ARTHRITIS

ARTHRITIS

Complete, Up-to-Date Facts
for Patients and Their Families

SHELDON PAUL BLAU, M.D.
AND DODI SCHULTZ

Doubleday & Company, Inc., Garden City, New York

1974

ISBN: 0-385-09476-0
LIBRARY OF CONGRESS CATALOG CARD NUMBER 73–81987

PRO

Ed, Bette (seniores priores),
Steven et Debra,
fide et amore

Joe
amicus et frater

Helen
sine cui non, a primo ad ultimum

Contents

Introduction

What is arthritis?

A television commercial of not too long ago would have us believe it is a minor ailment posing occasional problems for women of an uncertain—but certainly grandmotherly—age trying to tie bows on gift packages or manipulate the lids of cold-cream jars. And that a couple of pills or capsules, containing a mysterious ingredient "doctors recommend most," promise to banish the trouble in a trice.

The facts are a little different. At least fifty million Americans are afflicted to some extent by chronic arthritis, although many are unaware of it; almost 40 percent of those require medical care. A great many arthritis victims are elderly, but many are not; some, in fact, are children. The majority of its victims are probably female, but the proportion is by no means overwhelming; the best estimate is that about 45 percent of those severely afflicted by the major arthritic disorders are males (who constitute 49 percent of the U.S. population).

There is indeed one form that specifically strikes older persons—but it can begin as early as the twenties and, by and large, practices no sex discrimination. Another form does strike at least three times as many women as men—not in their declining years, but in the prime of life; 80 percent of its victims are un-

Arthritis

der the age of forty when the condition first appears. Still other
major forms are far more prevalent in men.

There are a number of chronic, continuing conditions characterized chiefly by arthritis. It also adds to the pain and discomfort of a number of *other* chronic diseases, playing a major role
in those sometimes quite serious afflictions. It can be caused by
injury, as well. And it can appear as a complication of many
infectious diseases, most familiarly—but by no means limited to
—rubella.

Arthritis is never, per se, fatal. Yet it represents a major medical problem in our country. It is America's number-three cause
of disability (after heart and circulatory disorders and mental illness). It is responsible for an annual loss of more than fourteen
million work days in business and industry, plus uncounted days
in other, nonremunerated pursuits such as ordinary housekeep-
ing—plus an estimated 1.5 *billion* hours of something loosely
called "reduced efficiency," meaning that the work gets done,
somehow, but not as well as it might. It generates a yearly
medical bill of one billion dollars—plus one billion, seven hundred million dollars in lost wages. It lies behind an estimated 12
percent of our welfare expenditures. The figures we have cited
are conservative. All in all, its total cost to our economy is believed to be in excess of nine billion dollars each year—an increase of more than 100 percent since the mid-1960s. Not to
mention the cost in human suffering.

Clearly, the message of the commercial was a misleading one.
Arthritis simply *isn't* a momentary twinge that can be dispelled
by a pill or two. And there's another dangerous facet to the
promotional picture: the encouragement of self-diagnosis, as
well as self-medication.

The medications so promoted are legitimate ones—for some
problems, sometimes including certain forms of arthritis. But

not necessarily in the forms and dosages suggested by the ads. And some types of arthritis, improperly or inadequately treated, can and do lead to serious deformity and crippling. Further, many *other* ills may *masquerade* as arthritis or include arthritis (or apparent arthritis) as an early symptom; some of these are critical conditions in which delay in skilled diagnosis and treatment can be at best risky, at worst fatal. One in three persons who seek out a specialist for arthritis treatment, in fact, is found to be actually suffering, basically, from another disorder; these have ranged from infections to malfunction of endocrine glands, from circulatory problems to malignancies—all of which require prompt treatment.

A third result of widespread misinformation or lack of information, and a tragic result in more ways than one, has been reliance by desperate victims of arthritis or supposed arthritis on worthless "remedies": on "magic rays" and "moon dust," on fad foods and copper bracelets, on unqualified quacks dispensing alleged "cures." One reason, as we've noted, has been self-diagnosis. Another has been the fact that science simply does not yet have all the answers. A third is the clear need for more physicians, both to care for arthritis victims and to seek new, effective therapies. Members of the American Rheumatism Association section of the Arthritis Foundation, the organization of physicians concerned with arthritis and related conditions— which includes not only rheumatologists (those specializing in treating such disorders) but internists, orthopedists, pediatricians, family physicians, and others with particular interest in the problem—number, at this writing, fewer than twenty-five hundred.

Tracking down new treatments and medications is a fairly costly activity. Training skilled specialists also requires substantial funds. A mere fifteen million dollars a year, according to the National Health Education Committee, is being spent for arthritis research, approximately two thirds of that sum by the National Institute of Arthritis and Metabolic Diseases in Washington, D.C. Those figures, the committee has pointed out, can be compared with these annual expenditures by Americans: fourteen billion dollars for liquor; eight billion dollars for tobacco and related products; more than two hundred and twenty million dollars for hair colorings. And, some *four hundred million dollars* on folk "remedies" and quack "cures."

Can you imagine what even a fraction of that four hundred million dollars might do in providing *real* help and hope for arthritics? We can. We hope, when you have finished reading this book, that you, too, will share our concern and dismay.

That is, however, not our primary purpose in writing it; it is not intended as an impassioned plea for financial aid to arthritis research and training, though we shall be delighted if that is one result. (As we have noted, the economic cost of arthritic disorders to our nation has doubled in the past decade. Federal support for arthritis research has, however, been at a virtual standstill, with an average increase of 2.8 percent a year, while the cost of living has soared at an annual rate of 3.6 percent— thus, in terms of dollar value of that support, reflecting a decrease in practical terms.) Researchers and clinical rheumatologists are needed desperately now, and the need grows more critical daily. We have pointed out that arthritis does affect more older (not necessarily elderly) people than younger ones; thus, as our life expectancy increases—and more and more people live longer and longer—the number of those afflicted with the varying forms of arthritis is bound to increase as well.

(A brief comment on the effect of those increased expectations might be in order. Life expectancy for a newborn baby in ancient Rome stood at a mere twenty-five or thirty years—a figure that had risen by the Middle Ages to thirty-three, by the latter part of the nineteenth century to more than forty, by 1900 to forty-seven. If you are a male born in 1920, your life expectancy at birth was fifty-four years; if you were born in 1940, sixty-one years; in 1960, sixty-seven years; the equivalent figures for females were fifty-five, sixty-five, and seventy-three years. Further, life expectancy grows by a small increment with each year of survival. A man born in 1930, for example, who survived until 1970, could then expect to live at least to the age of seventy-two, a woman to seventy-eight; someone who turned twenty in 1970 could look forward to a total of at least seventy years if male, seventy-seven if female. Yes, life expectancy for females is now substantially greater. In the decade between 1960 and 1970, the U.S. population increased 13 percent—but the number of those over sixty-five rose 20 percent, and of *women* over sixty-five, almost 30 percent. This final observation: in 1920, those Americans—male or female—who were at least sixty-five years old represented about *half* those who *might* have survived to that age; the current figures are 66 percent for males, 81 percent for females.)

Our *primary* reason for writing this book is to inform. Do *not* let it take the place of expert medical advice. If you have arthritis, we hope we will be able to give you a full picture of your illness, to present insights your physician may not have the time to spell out. If someone in your family has arthritis, we hope you will come away with a deeper understanding of what she or he may be suffering. If you *suspect* that you or someone close to you may have one of the arthritic disorders, we urge you to seek competent medical diagnosis—*not* to attempt such diagnosis on the basis of this book or any other, *or* on the basis of suggestions from your friendly neighborhood pharmacist.

Above all, we have made every effort to present here all the facets of the problem, both positive and negative—its promising aspects as well as the bluntly disappointing ones, the conquests and the continuing frustrations—in order to give you a picture that is both honest and lucid.

ONE

Defining Our Terms
(What Is Arthritis, Anyway?)

Sir James George Frazer, in his fascinating and deservedly famed study of worldwide folklore, The Golden Bough, tells of a quaint belief still extant—at least in the 1920s, when this now-classic work was first published—among certain natives of southeastern Australia. These tribesmen, he found, had concluded that the inexplicable pangs of arthritis were caused by some disgruntled foe who had stealthily followed them and placed bits of broken glass or other sharp fragments in their footprints! Similar beliefs have arisen in other parts of the world—perhaps not unrelated to the reliance, in certain cultures, on the causing of disease by the sticking of pins into wax images or other doll-like representations.

Silly? Maybe. But arthritis has been with man, so far as we can now tell, since the dawn of history and perhaps in prehistoric periods as well. (Clear evidence was found, for example, when Egyptian mummies were X-rayed for the first time in the late 1960s, that not even the royal figures who were to occupy the pyramids had escaped: Ramses the Second, for one, who ruled the kingdom of the Nile from 1304 to 1225 B.C., suffered from severe arthritis of the hip.) It is perhaps understandable that explanations, however illogical, were readily accepted; man has always had a penchant for explaining things, and if a logical cause cannot be found, any available one will frequently do. We still don't know everything, and we still do not have clear, rational explanations for some forms of arthritis—but as we'll see, we *have* gotten a bit beyond the broken-glass theory. Perhaps a good deal *more* than a bit.

To return to our question: what *is* this thing called arthritis? The terms you may have heard—and which are still used to one extent or another—are at best confusing. And you may not find your dictionary of much help. If you consult an older, but authoritative, one, you may find that *arthritis* was considered a synonym for *gout*. "Rheumatism," another term you may have heard and connected with our subject, was listed as a broad term enveloping stiffness and pain from whatever cause.

We might as well start with a comment on derivation; that often provides key clues. The "arthr-" part of arthritis and arthritic comes from the Greek word *arthron*—meaning, simply, joint. The "rheuma" part of rheumatism (or rheumatic, or rheumatoid) comes from another Greek word—*rheuma*, meaning a stream. *What* stream? Probably one of the "humors" the earliest physicians were wont to credit for all human ills; these were mysterious substances that flowed around the body, causing, by their presence or absence, a variety of inimical conditions. The first of these derivations is obviously far more precise than the second; nevertheless, both hand-me-downs have doggedly hung on—though today's usages are distinctly different from those of a generation ago.

What the Words Mean Now

So that we—and you—know precisely what we mean, we're going to set up our own definitions. In general, they reflect current medical thinking.

Arthritic diseases (or conditions, or disorders): those that involve arthritis as a major, or defining, symptom and are essentially chronic problems; also including some chronic joint conditions that are not essentially inflammatory in nature. They include, most prominently—in rough order of prevalence —osteoarthritis, rheumatoid arthritis, systemic lupus erythematosus, gout, psoriatic arthritis, ankylosing spondylitis, scleroderma, and dermatomyositis. These are the topics we'll be discussing in detail in this book; each will be defined and explained individually as we come to it.

Arthritis: literally, inflammation (all medical terms ending in "-itis" denote inflammation) of a joint or joints (although, as previously noted, not all the arthritic disorders involve inflammation—although *most* do). Arthritis is thus a descriptive term rather than one that defines a particular condition; it does not by itself imply any of the disorders mentioned in the preceding paragraph. It may not, in fact, be associated with any of them, but may result from, say, injury to a particular joint; it may also exist as a symptom accompanying some other condition, such as a systemic infection; it can sometimes appear as a side effect of certain medications, notably some anticonvulsants, contraceptives, and major tranquilizers.

Arthritis may, for instance, appear in association with rubella; some 30 to 40 percent of those who have had this infection, also known as "German measles," have experienced some arthritis. It is a fairly consistent accompaniment of rheumatic fever, a streptococcal infection; here the joint involvement is typically migratory—i.e., moving from one joint to another. It may also go along with such diverse infectious ills as hepatitis (of which it is sometimes the first symptom), gonorrhea (the arthritis can cripple permanently if the infection is not promptly treated), tuberculosis (about 4 percent of all cases include arthritis), meningitis, and ulcerative colitis (one study found

3

arthritis in 17 percent of the cases sampled). None of these are classed as "arthritic diseases," because the joints are not basically where the problem lies; further, the specific infectious agent, and its primary action, are known. When prompt therapy is directed to the basic problem, and that therapy is successful, the arthritis can generally be expected to depart as well. Thus arthritis related to infection *can be cured*—and it is the *only* kind that can be, so far, no matter what you may hear to the contrary. (Of course, arthritis induced by, or occurring as a side effect of, a drug or medication can also be halted by ceasing the administration of that agent.)

You will note that the foregoing are chiefly specific infections—primarily involving not a joint, but some other part of the body: the liver, the nervous system, the gastrointestinal tract, etc. While further exploration of the idea is outside the scope of this book, it's interesting to note in passing that sometimes arthritic manifestations appear very early in the development of cancer—notably in leukemia and in a small but significant proportion of malignancies involving the lungs and other structures in the chest. Some researchers feel that this phenomenon lends support to the theory of invasion by some as yet unidentified infectious agent or agents being at the root of malignant disease.

The association of arthritic symptoms with infections has also lent credence to the increasing feeling that some of the arthritic disorders themselves—rheumatoid arthritis, in particular—may in fact *be* systemic infections, and a number of findings tend to support that notion. We shall discuss some of those findings in later chapters.

Rheumatic diseases (*or conditions, or disorders*): generally, now, the arthritic disorders *plus* others involving tissues or structures in, around, or connected with the joints. (The phrase

4

has lost all connection with its Greek root, and has broadened considerably beyond the term "rheumatism.") This term might now be defined as *disorders primarily or prominently attacking the joints and/or their surrounding or supporting tissues.* Thus, the rheumatic disorders include, by current thinking, the arthritic diseases; bursitis (inflammation of a small cushioning sac within a joint—"tennis elbow" is one example); fibrositis (a nonspecific condition characterized by achiness and stiffness, often associated with emotional trauma or with generalized infections such as flu); myositis (inflammation specifically of muscle tissue); tendinitis (inflammation of a tendon); various other conditions, whether transient or chronic, involving deterioration or dysfunction of such tissues.

Rheumatism: a word perhaps best abandoned at this point, at least as a disease designation. In our grandparents' day, when names had not been assigned to some of the conditions we have mentioned, it was a term loosely applied to any aches or pains, especially in the elderly, that seemed to center around the joints, and were otherwise unexplained. In Great Britain, it is still often synonymous with arthritis. Here in the United States, it has fallen into disuse except in the name of the American Rheumatism Association—where it is equivalent to *rheumatology.*

Rheumatologist: a physician specializing in the treatment and/or study of the rheumatic diseases in general and the arthritic disorders in particular; i.e., in the field called *rheumatology.* The most skilled such individuals are certified in the specialty, technically a subspecialty of internal medicine, by the American Board of Internal Medicine. (The subspecialty was not officially recognized until recently; the first qualifying examinations were given late in 1972, and few physicians across the country have, at this writing, been Board-certified in rheumatology. Obviously, the patient seeking expert treatment for an arthritic disorder cannot yet count on finding one of these physicians around the corner. There are, however, many specializing in internal medicine or family practice who are skilled in dealing with these disorders. Diplomas from the various certifying boards, incidentally, are generally displayed in the doctor's office; they should at least be available upon inquiry.)

Some, we might note, have confused this area with the quite different medical specialty called *orthopedics*. The orthopedist is concerned with the development, integrity, and function of the bones and associated skeletal structures and the treatment —especially surgical and rehabilitative treatment—of injuries and deformities involving such structures. Thus such a specialist, while not dealing primarily with the rheumatic (chiefly systemic) diseases, may be called upon in situations in which orthopedic skills can help to restore function or correct deformity; orthopedic surgery is in fact playing an increasingly important role in this area, as we shall explain in later chapters.

Inflammation

We've used this word a number of times. This is as good a point as any to comment a bit further on its meaning and nature.

Classic medical texts traditionally present inflammation as a condition characterized by a quartet of characteristics easy for medical students to memorize: *rubor* (from the Latin for redness), *calor* (heat—and yes, the calorie is technically a unit of heat), *tumor* (swelling—not, as it is more narrowly applied, a growth), and *dolor* (pain).

Put in ordinary, familiar terms, here's what happens. There is an injury (as, for example, a bruise) or an assault by some foreign substance (let's say a virus on the mucous membrane of the nose). Capillaries in the affected area react initially by constricting, then within a very short time dilate, causing redness (*rubor*). Nearby white cells of the blood and lymph circulations, carrying antibodies (substances designed to fight the cause of the trouble), flow into the area, causing swelling (*tumor*) and, because of their concentration, pressure felt as pain (*dolor*). Depending upon the nature and intensity of the battle, calls for further defenses may be sent out generally—i.e., the body may be stimulated to rush further fighters to the area, and the defensive mechanism may even be systemic, encompassing the entire body; part of that further defense involves heat (*calor*), either localized or generalized in the form of fever.

The foregoing has been somewhat oversimplified, but, roughly, that is what goes on in any situation involving injury or invasion of the body by a foreign substance (including bacteria and viruses—or an incompatible transplanted organ). Among the factors active in the process are certain enzymes. Enzymes, generally speaking, are chemical catalysts of various biological processes; they work to trigger actions or interactions. Some enzymes act helpfully; it is an enzyme carried by the sperm, for example, that breaks down the coating of the egg cell to permit the sperm to penetrate. Others can be lethal. The venom of some poisonous snakes, for instance, contains an enzyme called lecithinase (all enzyme names end in "-ase") that shatters red blood cells by attacking a part of their structure.

The enzymes active in the inflammation process come from within the body's cells, where they are contained in units called

7

lysosomes. When they are needed—e.g., to attack invading bacteria—their "cage," the lysosomal membrane, breaks down and they are unleashed to play their part in the defense effort. But in certain conditions, among them rheumatoid arthritis and some of the other arthritic diseases, the body's defensive batteries begin to attack the very cells of the body itself! We do not yet understand just how or why this occurs, but it is the reason you may hear these conditions referred to as *autoimmune disorders*—that is, disorders in which the body's defenses behave as if the body itself were an invading substance and become self-destructive.

Anti-Inflammation

Since inflammation figures prominently in most of the conditions we are going to discuss in this book, much research has centered on an effort to determine precisely how it works and what substances might block what is here a distinctly unhelpful frenzy of activity—as well as its accompanying pain. Aspirin is the most familiar of those substances; hence it is a basic therapy in just about all forms of arthritis. Cortisone and similar medications—adrenal hormones and synthetic versions of them—have also been found helpful to a degree; they seem to strengthen the lysosomal membranes, thus inhibiting the release of trouble-triggering enzymes. Other drugs have played a part as well, such as those known to suppress the body's "immune reactions"; these are the same sorts of drugs generally used to stave off rejection of transplanted organs.

None of these drugs is ideal; none is without its dangers. But we'll go into more detail about them, and their known effects both for good and for ill, when we come to discussion of the various specific disorders.

Defining Our Terms

Before we do that, let's take a look—for your amusement and, we hope, enlightenment—at some forms of arthritis "treatment" that are unqualifiedly hazardous and offer no redeeming features at all: folk "remedies" and quack "cures."

TWO

Fads, Fancies, &
the $400,000,000 Misunderstanding

Every disease and disorder known to man—and woman—has had its lore of miraculous "remedies" and "cures." Arthritis, which has plagued the human race since the dawn of history, is no exception. Some of the "prescriptions" arose from simple, primitive ignorance; others stemmed from early efforts to arrive at a scientific approach to disease and treatment; still others have been foisted upon the unwary sufferer by outright charlatans and profiteers. Many have found their way around the world, sometimes across oceans and centuries.

Here, a brief glimpse of just a few of these curiosities, past and present.

"Take My Arthritis—Please!"

One of the quaintest and most ancient of cures—and one of the few that haven't persisted in some form to the present—was the theory of transference, which was known (or perhaps traveled) from the Middle East to northern Europe. One could, so the theory went, "transfer" a disease or discomfort to some other living thing, if one knew the secret.

The guinea pig, for example, was thought to be an ideal

recipient for the aches of arthritis of almost any type; the "transference" could be accomplished just by keeping one of the creatures in one's home overnight. By morning the hapless animal would be suffering, its host fully recovered. But usually, things weren't quite so simple—as illustrated by two specific gout prescriptions that have come down to us, both "transferring" the condition to trees.

One such formula involved a fir tree, the younger and suppler the better. The transfer tactic was simply to tie a knot in one of the tree's twigs, while reciting: "God greet thee, noble fir. I bring thee my gout. Here will I tie a knot and bind my gout into it." If that did not produce results, it was, we assume, repeated until a more receptive tree was found.

A second ritual required an oak tree and was a little more complicated. The sufferer's nails were trimmed and a few hairs clipped from his legs; then both nail parings and hairs were placed in a small hole bored in the tree and the hole sealed with cow dung. A three-month gout-free period was "proof" that the condition had been successfully transferred to the tree. As it happens, an acute attack of gout is very likely to disappear within days or weeks, and unlikely to recur within three months —so this remedy was pretty much a sure thing.

From Rome, with Faith

A number of beliefs—both in remedies and in charms to "ward off" arthritic attacks—can be traced back to notions of the ancient Greeks and Romans. Some of them have survived to this very day, and in this very country.

One was a belief in the mysterious curative powers of certain metals. The earliest of these, so far as we know, was copper. At Bath, in England, excavation of a Roman spa, dating from the days when the Romans ruled the British Isles as well as the rest of Europe, revealed the source of the still-popular superstition concerning the copper bracelet as a protective device.

The waters of the mineral spring there, it seems, were believed to have special curative powers. Custom dictated that those arthritics who had been "cured" by immersion in the baths, in gratitude to the gods for that benevolent gesture, anchor to a wall of the baths a copper bracelet bearing the name of the now-healthy supplicant. An additional—and powerful—element was thought to enter into the waters as they lapped at the bracelets set firmly in the walls; thus, each bracelet would add to the efficacy of the baths for succeeding sufferers. Many of the bracelets, still firmly anchored and apparently whole and undissolved, can still be seen by visitors to the excavation site.

Perhaps derived from that early influence was a custom that arose in England quite a bit later, and continued through the mid-sixteenth-century reign of Queen Mary I. Each Good Friday, arthritis sufferers appeared before the ruling monarch and presented for royal blessing rings fashioned from metal—usually silver, iron, or brass—that had been used on a coffin. That blessing was believed to bestow healing power, and the ring became a potent "remedy" for its wearer's ills.

Unaccountably, the metallic-magic belief has kept recurring. The still-extant belief in the warding-off powers of copper is well-known; it has taken the form not only of bracelets, but of shoes studded with copper nails. As a switch on that, some have a specific faith in zinc. In Appalachia, a belief in the power of a magnet to "draw the pain out" is said to persist—and in some other areas, a trust in "magnetic" belts and rings.

Another derivation from ancient beliefs is the charm—the

amulet that would, by a special power it possessed, shield the bearer from evil. The belief certainly existed in Egypt, and it was probably passed on as contacts between peoples progressed. We do know that the Greeks believed all ills were caused by wandering evil spirits—an idea espoused by the greatest of their philosophers, such as Aristotle; the more educated knew that there was some physical process involved, but surmised that those malevolent spirits set the disease-causing "humors" flowing to do their damage. Among such charms still wistfully believed by some folk in the Old World and the New to prevent or ward off "rheumatism" (all, to be carried in the pocket): a potato (it's sometimes specified that it must be peeled and kept until it turns black); buckshot; nutmegs; horse chestnuts; the right forefoot of a rabbit; the foot of a mole, selected to reflect the site of the sufferer's affliction.

Still another early influence, espoused by such prominent writers as the first-century A.D. Roman naturalist Pliny the Elder, was the curing of disorders by applying some specific object or substance externally to the troubled area. Sometimes such prescriptions were wholly magical, involving incantations, the twining of ribbons in a certain way, the laying on of mosses gathered at midnight by the light of a full moon, and the like. Often, the materials were animal or vegetable, and an elastic imagination contrived some relationship between the disease and its "cure."

Thus the rheumatic diseases, with their accompanying stiffness, came to be associated with cold—quite logically to be countered by "hot" substances. Garlic was an old European favorite that found its way to other climes as well—though by the time it reached India, the prescription took the form of frying the garlic, then rubbing the afflicted joint with the pungent oil, rather than with the herb itself. In the East Indies, the substance employed was Spanish pepper—to be rubbed, curiously, not on the trouble site, but into the fingernails and toenails.

Animal substances typically took the major character of the beast itself into account. Those championed for arthritis have come from the most supple animals—most prominently, and not surprisingly, the snake; its oils were long believed to impart new flexibility to joints on which they were applied. (It must be added, though, that some of the "snake oil" liniments promoted during the nineteenth-century patent-medicine heyday —of which, more shortly—contained not a drop of reptilian oil, but were compounded chiefly of camphor, kerosene, turpentine, and the like.) In the Americas, the fat of graceful felines has been favored—notably the wildcat in rural areas of the United States, the mountain lion in the Sierra Madre region of Mexico.

A Potpourri of Foods and Folk Potions

When it comes to internal remedies for the rheumatic disorders, the list is virtually endless; we could probably fill an entire book with a recitation of all the concoctions that have been dreamed up over the years. They have included practically every herb from celery seed to garlic to henbane. Sarsaparilla and comfrey had their day, as did yucca plants and pokeberries, lilies, thistles, alfalfa, barley, rhubarb, and the barks and saps of trees. Many of the prescriptions have very practically included dissolving the "medicine" in such conveniently pain-obliterating liquids as wine or whiskey; "white lightning" moonshine has been a favorite vehicle among some backwoods devotees of such fancies in our own part of the world.

Such ideas have by no means been limited to the backwoods, however; many, as you may be aware, have spread among presumably knowledgeable and sophisticated city folk, as well.

Significantly, in recent years they are often associated not with a natural substance, but with a packaged product handily available at the nearest drugstore or supermarket.

Certain fruits came into vogue in the 1950s, notably canned cherries. Later, orange juice became the fad—followed more recently by massive doses of vitamin C (replaced in some avant-garde circles by vitamin E or more esoteric "health foods").

Sometimes such nonsense has actually been encouraged—even promoted—by presumed medical authorities, often with elaborate explanations. One example was the infamous honey-and-vinegar hoax of the early 1960s. Its advocates claimed curative powers for this unsavory potion based on the totally erroneous premise that arthritis stems from a combination of chunks of pure calcium lodged in the joints with an "alkaline" condition—and that vinegar (the honey was presumably present to make it a bit more palatable) would "dissolve" the calcium and, being acid, neutralize the "alkalinity."

It's interesting to note that another "remedy" later advocated on the medical fringe, a decoction of the Chinese herb ginseng, was sworn to "work" because it neutralized the "excess acid" that flowed into the joints and "caused inflammation." (A type of acid secretion is involved in one form of arthritis, gout, but the "remedy" was recommended for all the rheumatic disorders.)

Secrets of the Noble Red Man

No survey of folk remedies would be complete without mention of the colorful patent-medicine industry that flowered in the United States during the last decades of the nineteenth century. The "medicines" were generally fairly innocuous, pills and "tonics" adapted from old folk remedies or concocted by aspiring entrepreneurs in back rooms of small shops. The results were then heavily promoted—by smaller operators from the backs of traveling carnival wagons, by larger firms via posters, circulars, and splashy ads in newspapers, magazines, and almanacs. The advertising was often quite inventive, outdoing —in those days prior to governmental regulation of drug promotion—anything the modern Madison Avenue imagination could conjecture.

One of the most prominent outfits—which will serve as a typical example of this peculiarly American phenomenon—was the Comstock clan, which was active in the business under a variety of names and under the aegis of different members of the family for over a century, starting in the 1830s. Their products were marketed not only throughout the United States and Canada, but in England, Australia, and the Orient as well. Carlton's Liniment, occasionally dubbed Carlton's Nerve & Bone Liniment, one of the standbys of its broad-ranging line of "celebrated medicines" for man and beast, actually began as a rubdown for horses, but by the 1850s had somehow become a medicine for humans and was proclaimed a "certain remedy" not merely for rheumatism, but for burns, bruises, sores, sprains, and piles! (In the company's last days—its doors finally closed in 1960—under far more stringent federal curbs, the product, renamed Comstock's N & B Liniment, was purveyed simply as a "powerful counterirritant," which it probably was, for the relief of "muscular pains" and similar conditions, and the relief was carefully described as temporary.)

Many of the promotional schemes for the patent medicines involved claims that the origins of the remedies were mysterious or exotic, suggestions that seemed to enhance their appeal to the public. One such was another Comstock concoction,

Longley's Great Western Indian Panacea, which allegedly possessed curative powers encompassing practically all known ills. It was a sure cure for chronic rheumatism *and*, its label promised, "Asthma, Dispepsia, Coughs, Colds and all Scrofula and other Diseases arising from an impure State of the Blood and all Kidney and Liver Complaints"—adding that "as a family physic it is unequalled."

A sumptuously illustrated sales pitch on the wrapper implied that the Panacea was a miraculous natural substance discovered by Indian medicine men, or, as the label had it, "The rude sons of nature a medicine find,/That heals all diseases which trouble mankind." One wonders why the firm felt it necessary to offer any *other* products for sale!

But offer they did, and by far the most famous item in their pharmacopoeia was Dr. Morse's Indian Root Pills. The efficacy of this remedy reached even beyond that of the "panacea," for the pills were claimed able to banish not only rheumatism, but a host of ills including headache, constipation, piles, boils, colds, malaria, eczema, worms, "female complaints," neuralgia, "la grippe," kidney disease, palpitation, and bad breath. The promotional story that went with them related in exciting detail how "Dr. Morse" had obtained the secret remedy while traveling among the Indians of the wild West, returning from his journeys just in time to restore his aged, rapidly expiring father to robust health. There was, of course, no Dr. Morse; the pills were compounded by a New York chemist named Moore, who was subsequently bought out by the Comstocks. (Anything omitted from the list of indications for the "Indian root" pills was covered by claims for a companion product, Judson's Mountain Herb Pills, promoted as an ancient healing formula of the Aztecs confided to one "Dr. Cunard"—who was just as fictitious as Dr. Morse.)

The ingredients of the "root" pills were of course kept extremely secret. But federal law changed all that, and the label finally listed the components. At least in their last days of U.S. manufacture—the 1940s and 1950s—the pills contained aloes (a laxative), mandrake (traditionally touted as an "aphrodisiac"), gamboge (a gum from a tree of the Far East, sometimes used there as a cathartic), jalap (the root of a Mexican plant and another powerful purgative), and cayenne pepper, with some sugar thrown in to improve the taste. In those last years, too, advertising for the pills abandoned the fantastic claims and presented the stuff for what it was, a laxative—though probably not "mild and gentle," as the ads promised.

The "Indian root" pills, incidentally, despite the demise of the Comstock operation here, are still being made and sold at this writing by a branch of the company yet surviving in Australia (originally a subsidiary of the Canadian firm; the Comstocks had incorporated there as well as in the United States), but as a laxative, nothing more.

Yet while the patent-medicine boom is now a thing of the past, promoters of the Comstock ilk still surface from time to time, hoping to take profitable advantage of the ill and ignorant. In late 1972, the federal government, in a postal service seizure action, confiscated a quantity of "Chaparral Herb Tablets"—claimed effective not only for treatment of arthritis, but of leprosy, cancer, and venereal disease as well!

Magic Rays, Moon Dust, and Other Modern Mumbo Jumbo

In these days of space travel and transplanted hearts, arthritis sufferers familiar through their newspapers and television screens with up-to-the-minute details of scientific advance are a good deal less likely to fall for such stuff as magical herbs, moles' feet, and healing lore of the ancient Aztecs. Yet it is, perhaps, precisely *because* the previously incredible—men walking about on the surface of the moon, one man's heart beating in the breast of another—has become credible, that doubt can still be suspended. *Anything* is, perhaps, possible. The *new* magic is science itself.

Thus some who would look with disdain on a nutmeg in the pocket or a copper bracelet on the wrist have been ready to trust the claims of those promoting the benefits of lamps emitting "healing rays"; of radiations from uranium ore; of the curative effects of powdery fragments brought back from the moon (analysis of the "moon dust" actually purveyed for a time after the astronauts' first flight revealed it to be quite ordinary dust, of strictly earthly origin).

Thus, too, it has been possible for unscrupulous "medical" practitioners to persuade the credulous that they have by "scientific" means come upon therapies and treatments that are simply not acceptable to "vested interests" in the medical and pharmaceutical "establishment."

Even a few real physicians, with medical degrees, have been known to espouse and advertise pseudoscientific chemical "cures" for arthritis, claiming—whether due to sheer avarice or to mental aberration—victory through "research," dismissing doubters as jealous of their insights or discoveries. Perhaps because U.S. laws are designed to protect us in spite of our credulous selves, many such individuals can be found perched just over the Mexican or Canadian border, where neither their methods nor materials can be subjected to inspection by American authorities, but where they are easily reached by American clientele. Their "medicines" range from worthless to potentially lethal; one such "cure," reported in 1971 and possibly still being administered by a private practitioner in Montreal, involved potentially hazardous blends of sex hormones and other endocrine drugs, along with diuretics and a variety of irrelevant vitamins.

Why the Kooks and Quacks Survive

As we noted in our introduction, Americans who have arthritis (or who *believe* they have arthritis) are estimated to spend some $400,000,000—*four hundred million dollars*—every single year on fake "cures," bizarre "remedies," and innumerable gimmicks that are totally worthless.

Some are hazardous per se. *All* are dangerous in that they (1) divert money from the hands of those who have better uses for it into the pockets of quacks, con artists, and assorted charlatans; (2) substitute useless measures for real medical care, thus permitting the disease to continue uncontrolled and often leading to crippling that could have been prevented; (3) delay diagnosis, in many instances, of an acute, *non*arthritic condition that might have been totally cured had it been discovered but might, with time and without treatment, maim and even kill.

Why have arthritis sufferers so often fallen prey to such cruel hoaxes? Why have the perpetrators of the frauds found it so easy to turn up new lambs to fleece?

There are probably several reasons, some applying in other kinds of disorders as well.

—Some disorders cannot yet be truly cured. If someone has— or *thinks* he or she has—a condition that simply cannot be cured by any legitimate means known to medicine, that individual is often a ready foil for practitioners claiming to have discovered a "cure" that conventional authorities do not accept. It is easy, if one is eager enough to believe, that "the AMA and the big drug companies" would rather perpetuate

suffering than concede the great "genius" of the "scientist" making the claims.

Of course this is simply not true. Any major drug manufacturer would give its eyeteeth to lay hands on a sure cure for arthritis, cancer, or anything else, and would unquestionably be delighted to cut its discoverer in on a share of the certainly huge profits. And doctors would hardly be thrown out of business; they would not want for patients if sure cures for cancer, arthritis, and the common cold were discovered tomorrow.

–*Some problems are not what the person who is ill believes them to be.* Let's say, for example, that Mrs. A's elbow hurts. She may have rheumatoid arthritis. She may have a bone tumor. She may have bursitis. She may have a sprain, or a pulled muscle, or an ordinary bruise. She may have nothing physical at all; there are such things as pains of purely psychogenic origin. She doesn't visit a physician to have the trouble diagnosed—but a friend convinces her that she is suffering from arthritis, and that she should visit "Doctor X," who is the sole possessor of the only cure in the world.

Doctor X provides her with a bottle of pills and assures her that her discomfort will vanish. She duly takes the pills as directed and lo, the pain in her elbow disappears! Maybe because she just *believed* it would. Maybe because it resulted from an injury, and was healed by time. Maybe because the condition—whatever it may be—has entered a pain-free phase. But Mrs. A believes that she had arthritis, and that it was cured. And Doctor X has acquired another walking advertisement.

–*Chronology is confused with cause and effect.* Here lies the dividing line between superstition and rational science. Superstition, noting the order in time of events, postulates that the earlier caused the later: thus the fork that was dropped before the guest arrived, the black cat seen before the turn of ill luck, the penny found before the pleasant stroke of chance become the direct *causes* of the events that follow. It is easy to proceed from there to the connection between the copper bracelet and the absence of pain, or the pill taken and the disappearance of discomfort. It is of course just as easy to draw any of a number of other conclusions, since one is perfectly free, by this means, to decide that a disorder may be avoided or cured by dialing the telephone with one's third finger, by drinking a martini every other Tuesday, or by running backward three times around the block.

True therapies are arrived at far differently. They are tested and retested not by one researcher but by many. Objective rather than subjective criteria are used. Comparisons are made with other materials and other methods, to eliminate even the possibility of inadvertently drawing wrong conclusions.

—Spontaneous remission can occur. Physicians have learned to be wary of conclusion-leaping, particularly in the arthritic disorders, because of their variety of causes and patterns. As we noted earlier, arthritis can occur in association with infectious ills such as rubella. That sort of arthritis generally persists for a period of days or weeks, but it does disappear eventually—whether there is any treatment or not; it is what is called *self-limited*, and the remission is permanent.

Some major kinds of arthritis are indeed chronic—i.e., continu*ing*—but are discontinu*ous*; rheumatoid arthritis is one example. Such disorders follow a flare-and-remission pattern that is unpredictable. Thus quacks have convinced their victims that a "cure" has been achieved when the disease goes into a quiescent period—while a legitimate physician who is treating the condition knows (and will let the patient know) that it is likely to return at a later date; here the remission is temporary.

Perhaps you have never once considered the sort of "treatments" we've talked about in this chapter; if that's so, we're glad. But if you have, we hope you now have some new insights into human gullibility—and where it can lead.

In the chapters that follow, we shall share with you what is known of the actual causes of, and valid remedies for, the chronic arthritic diseases.

THREE

All This and Arthritis Too:
The Collagen Diseases

This subclassification of the arthritic disorders is fortunately a small one, for the conditions it covers are quite serious—and they are also among the most mystifying in all of rheumatology. If you or someone you know has been diagnosed as a victim of one of them, and the physician seems vague about treatment, it's not because he or she is ill-informed or uneducated; it's because there is so little definitive information available.

What *is* a "collagen disease"?

Collagen is a protein substance that forms an important part of connective tissue fibrils of all sorts—not only in the joints, but throughout the body. In the collagen diseases, any of the connective tissues may be affected. Because many such tissues *are* associated with the joints, typically arthritis—that is, joint involvement—*is* a prominent part of the picture.

There are a great number of these uncommon disorders. Those that have been seen most often, and about which most is known—although it is still precious little—are systemic lupus erythematosus (frequently shortened to SLE), dermatomyositis, and scleroderma. Exact figures are not known, but SLE is probably ten times as prevalent as the other two combined.

Rheumatoid arthritis is sometimes categorized as a "collagen disease" as well, since it does affect connective tissue. Further, there are certain other diagnostic similarities—as well as the fact that rheumatoid arthritis, like the conditions we cover in this chapter, afflicts more women than men. But because rheumatoid arthritis attacks the joints almost exclusively while these three typically exhibit various symptoms, among which joint discomfort is not necessarily the most prominent, we think it makes a good deal more sense to consider them separately.

Systemic Lupus Erythematosus (SLE)

"Lupus" is a family name for a number of different conditions stemming from a variety of causes, all to some extent involving the skin. Sometimes the word alone has been used to mean one such condition, but that's like using the word "arthritis"; it doesn't really spell out which disorder is under discussion. *Lupus mutilans, lupus tumidus,* and *lupus vulgaris,* for instance, are three of a number of names for cutaneous tuberculosis—a skin condition known to be caused by the tuberculosis bacillus.

There are, in fact, two forms of lupus erythematosus (*erythema* derives from the Greek for "redness"): discoid lupus erythematosus (DLE) and systemic lupus erythematosus (SLE). In the first, so-called because of the roughly disc-shaped lesions that appear on the skin, *only* the skin is affected; SLE, as we've said, can affect connective tissues throughout the body, whether in the skin, joints, or elsewhere.

Some half a million to a million Americans are afflicted with SLE. Of every thirty victims, at least twenty, probably closer to twenty-five or twenty-six, are female—i.e., the ratio may be as high as five to one. Though it tends to strike during young adulthood, prominently during the two decades from the age of twenty to the age of forty, that's just an average, and not true in every single case; the youngest patient on record, at this writing, was only two years old, the oldest ninety-seven. But the advent of SLE after the age of sixty is considered extremely rare; it has been estimated that of all women with SLE, onset after age sixty has occurred in fewer than 10 percent.

Symptoms of SLE are extremely variable; underlying them all is that mysterious process in which the body seems to be irrationally attacking itself, with the inflammatory action we talked about in Chapter 1 surfacing almost anywhere. Slightly more than half of all SLE patients present—that's short for show-up-at-the-doctor's-office—with a certain amount of joint pain or discomfort, similar to that of rheumatoid arthritis but typically milder; often, as in the latter condition, there are complaints of early-morning stiffness in particular. Nine out of ten SLE victims will have accompanying arthritis sooner or later.

The first symptoms in another 15 to 25 percent are cutaneous, involving the skin—usually *not* anywhere near the joints. Very often this is a reddish rash that occurs especially in areas exposed to the sun, such as the face and hands. A classic sign of SLE, in fact, is a "butterfly" rash that extends over the bridge of the nose, its "wings" arcing out over the cheekbones on each side. Such a rash—whether it assumes a "butterfly" shape or not—occurs in at least 75 percent of SLE cases sooner or later, and in over a third it *is* the "butterfly" type; it may take the form of shiny lumps in the affected area, or simple reddening—often, only upon exposure to sunlight.

The third early symptom is usually fever, another possibly significant hint for researchers, which in most SLE patients accompanies whatever other symptoms may be present.

Thus far, SLE does not sound terribly serious. Fever, initially —plus mild joint pains, maybe, or perhaps a moderately annoying rash or redness. But it is other parts of the body, basically, with which we are most concerned. Any body tissue whatever may be affected. Extreme weakness may occur, as may anemia. Muscles, tendons, and such organs as the kidneys can be involved, and when that happens, there is quite a serious problem. The kidneys are instrumental in the body's continuing disposal of waste materials. That disposal is vital to the continuing viability of all the body's systems, bar none. There are such things as kidney transplants; but they often do not "take" under normal circumstances, and in SLE, there is a very *high* possibility of rejection.

To top all this off, SLE has another baffling characteristic in common with rheumatoid arthritis: it may be intermittent— coming and going. When it goes, there is no predicting, with assurance, when and where it will return. All we are sure of is there is a strong probability that it *will* return.

Diagnosis of SLE is by no means impossible, but it can be rather tricky. As with a number of other arthritic disorders, the pattern of the disease is so variable that symptoms experienced by one individual may be totally different from those of another. As with many of the arthritic disorders, however, the American Rheumatism Association has established valuable guidelines in the form of specific diagnostic criteria; they include both clinical observations and sophisticated laboratory techniques.

There are at this writing no less than fourteen distinct signs of SLE. Among factors considered highly significant, and which the physician will consider: the pattern of the accompanying rash (if a rash is present); the nature of any skin lesions, determined by biopsy and laboratory analysis; the characteristic arthritic symptoms; the presence of certain proteins in the urine; the discovery of specific types of cells (called LE cells), as well as certain other telltale elements, in blood samples drawn for chemical analysis. A definite diagnosis of SLE demands that at least four clear manifestations, out of that possible fourteen, be present.

No one, as we've said, knows the exact cause of SLE. But there have been a number of very intriguing clues, to wit:

—Cells incorporating viruslike particles have been isolated and cultured from SLE sufferers—even from samples of skin unaffected by the disease. They seem to be most like the paramyxoviruses, a particular class of viruses similar to—but differing in significant ways from—those that cause the various kinds of flu. The paramyxoviruses cause, among other things, the parainfluenzas (a group of relatively minor respiratory infections) and mumps. Fever, which typifies systemic infections, usually accompanies SLE at the start.

Is SLE an infectious disease?

—SLE victims often possess an extraordinary level of antibodies to a number of known viruses, among them those known to cause measles and the major types of flu. Antibodies to particular infectious organisms are produced by the body not at random, but only in response to attack by those organisms; their presence thus indicates such an attack, past or present. It is already known that certain viruses are capable of causing more than one kind of trouble in the same individual at different times. One such virus goes by the name of *Herpesvirus varicellae*; if you encounter this virus, you may come down with the ailment medically termed varicella, commonly known as chickenpox. If, having had chickenpox, you again encounter the same virus later in life, you will not have chickenpox again but you *may* be struck by quite another condition: herpes zoster, better known as shingles. The second encounter seems to reactivate, or "reawaken," the virus's potential for making mischief.

There are also a number of ailments that have been pegged to "slow-virus" causation, or in which there is strong evidence for such a suspicion. They are, thus far, chiefly ills of the nervous system. One is Parkinsonism, which has been almost surely traced to a 1920s epidemic of encephalitis. Another is a rare disease called subacute (chronic and progressive) sclerosing (gradually hardening) panencephalitis (brain inflammation) —SSPE, for short; the agent is the measles virus, or something microscopically indistinguishable from it. A third condition in which such a cause is postulated is multiple sclerosis, and the culprit suspected at this writing is, interestingly, one of the paramyxovirus type.

The pattern suggested in these situations is that the viral agent, instead of behaving in its usual manner, finds its way to some other part of the body and lies dormant for a period of years or even decades—what might be called an abnormal "incubation period." Such viral patterns have already been demonstrated conclusively in some animal ailments, including a disease of sheep called scrapie and an affliction of certain breeds of mink, which attacks the liver and kidney and also includes symptoms much like human arthritis.

Might SLE be triggered by a known virus—either by reactivation or by that delayed-action mechanism?

–SLE victims seem to have an unusually high incidence of allergies to chemical substances—penicillin, for example—as compared with the general population. Allergies, it is well known, often occur multiply rather than singly. We can have allergic responses to anything—not only pollens or house dust, medications or strawberries or peanuts, but to disease-causing organisms as well; rheumatic fever, for example, is now thought of medically as a hypersensitive response to streptococcus (or to its chemical by-products)—an organism that normally causes nothing more than a sore throat or, at worst, scarlet fever. In SLE there is a clear fight-off-the-invader sort of activity going on—except that no one has yet seen that "invader," and the effort seems to have a boomerang effect.

Could it be that SLE is an allergic response—either to a virus or other infectious agent, or to some substance not as yet recognized?

—We know that SLE can be—and, in fact, has been—induced by certain drugs, prominently hydralazine (Apresoline), which is used in treatment of high blood pressure; procainamide (Pronestyl), a drug used to control cardiac arrythmias (abnormal heartbeat rhythms); and, on occasion, various antibiotics, major tranquilizers (phenothiazines), and other medications.

Such instances are rare (i.e., taking one of these drugs by no means entails a high risk of SLE). And significantly, in such cases—unlike the "spontaneous" sort of SLE—the condition is wholly reversible; cutting off the medication stops the SLE cold. There are also two other distinguishing characteristics. Drug-induced SLE displays no sex bias; it afflicts as many men as women. And in the drug-induced form there is rarely involvement of either the kidneys or the central nervous system.

It is strongly suspected that this phenomenon represents some type of allergic response. Again, the question: might "spontaneous" SLE also be caused by allergy?

—Statistics suggest that there may be an increasing incidence of SLE, notes the Arthritis Foundation—although, the foundation adds, improved diagnosis could well result in a greater number of recorded cases, thus an *apparent* increase. But if the increase is a true one, that opens another avenue of thought. It is a known fact that certain familial ills, such as cystic fibrosis and diabetes, are actually becoming more widespread. The reason is that modern medicine can now control them so that they are no longer inevitably fatal (as they once were); hence, those suffering from them survive to pass on the applicable traits to their offspring. Perhaps a similar phenomenon is taking place with SLE.

Is SLE—or a susceptibility to it—inherited genetically? (If there is a hereditary component in SLE, it must be a fairly unusual one. SLE is more prevalent in females by a ratio of at least two to one, possibly as heavy as five to one—a far heavier proportion than in other known sex-linked hereditary traits. It should also be noted that, although some multiple occurrences among relatives have been reported, there is no clear evidence that SLE follows direct familial lines.) *

—If SLE, or a susceptibility to it, isn't hereditary, and whether the proximate cause is a virus, an allergen, or something else— there's still that unbalanced sex ratio to consider. Many medical theorists believe that certain of the female hormones serve to protect women in some way, to some extent, from some ills more prevalent among men, notably heart disease and a few kinds of cancer; these ills seem to attack women chiefly after the menopause. (Both sexes, by the way, produce both kinds of hormones; what makes men men and women women is a matter of which predominate.) Thus we might wonder if that sometimes works in reverse.

Does the clear prevalence of SLE among women, especially women of child-bearing age, bear some relationship to the

* Readers further interested in this subject will find it skillfully and lucidly explored in Amram Scheinfeld's *Heredity in Humans* (Lippincott, 1972).

female hormones—perhaps interacting, under special circumstances, with some other causative agent?

All of the preceding is, of course, sheer speculation at this point, despite the encouraging "hard" evidence in some areas. But it will give you some idea of the sort of painstaking detective work that medical research demands. Each such hypothesis must be tracked down, questioned, proved and reproved again and again. It is likely—even if the theory postulating an infectious agent ultimately proves true—to take a long time to pinpoint the precise viral villain, let alone specific therapy or prevention.

In the meantime, however, medicine *can* help the victim of SLE. But since symptoms vary so tremendously, treatment is necessarily highly individualized, geared to the needs of the particular patient at any particular time (that's true, too, of the other arthritic disorders). Of course there is frequent monitoring of the patient's condition through observation by both patient and doctor, and by laboratory tests as well.

Generally, SLE patients will be advised to avoid sunlight, since that may bring on symptoms or make them worse. Prolonged exposure to extreme cold can also sometimes produce the same effect. For the same reason, the doctor will usually warn against taking medications other than those prescribed, since they may by their action or interaction create undesirable effects. Strains on the system, whether physical or emotional—including undue fatigue, stressful situations, preventable infections, and injuries—are also best avoided.

How about medications? Nothing has been found, we reemphasize, that can be said to *cure* SLE. But there *are* a number of drugs of different types that can help to control the disease, relieve its symptoms, and in general strengthen the body's resistance to its ravages. And if you know someone who was treated for SLE some years back, know now that the therapeutic picture has changed a good deal in the last twenty or twenty-five years.

With the World War II discovery that drugs originally developed for the treatment of malaria also seemed to have a salutary effect in SLE, therapeutic emphasis over the next two decades centered on quinine derivatives, notably quinacrine (Atabrine) and chloroquine (Aralen), later a variation called hydroxychloroquine (Plaquenil) that proved a bit more desirable in terms of toxicity, but not much. The use of the quinine derivatives in treatment of SLE is now limited.

The trouble with the chloroquines is that they have a relatively high risk-to-benefit ratio. For one thing, there are such temporary but distressing side effects as graying hair and hair and nail loss. For another, they may interact in disturbing ways with such ubiquitous substances as antacids, alcohol, asthma medications, and certain analgesics. For a third, they are capable in rare—but nonetheless significant—instances of causing two types of eye problems: one, reversible after the medication is stopped, stemming from deposits within the eyeball; the other, resulting from degenerative changes in the retina—and *not* reversible. For these reasons, they are now considered useful only in treating, specifically, SLE rashes and joint involvement—and they are administered only with periodic eye examination.

Currently, three classes of drugs predominate in the treatment of SLE.

One is the very large group of anti-inflammatory substances and analgesics (pain relievers)—some of which act in *both* ways—including at one end of the spectrum such simple over-the-counter products as aspirin (an *extremely* useful drug), at the other vastly more complex and potent medications that can be obtained only by prescription.

The second is the corticosteroids—adrenal hormones and their synthetic and semisynthetic versions—that have the effect of helping the body cope with a number of conditions that have posed therapeutic problems in medicine.

Both these classes of drugs, because they are employed to one extent or another in almost all the arthritic disorders, are discussed in detail in Chapter 7.

The third kind of drug that has been proving especially useful in SLE is something we refer to, for lack of a more precise term, as an *immunosuppressive*. If you have read something about these drugs, it is probably in connection with transplant operations—the surgical transfer of organs such as the heart, lung, liver, or kidney from one individual to another. Typically, the human body will rear up and reject such alien organs; they are, it senses, "foreign," and they do not "belong."

The immunosuppressives specifically mute such reactions— in the case of a transplant, enabling the organ (hopefully) to "take hold" and "convince" the native tissue that it does indeed belong and is there to play a helpful, and even vital, role. If you *have* read about this, you also know the major drawback of these medications: they may also suppress the body's defensive responses to things it *ought* to be booting out, such as disease-causing organisms. Which means that whatever they're used for, they have to be used very, very carefully, to say the least.

What are the names of these drugs, and how do they work? The first part of the question is easy to answer. The chief ones, as this is written, are azathioprine (Imuran), cyclophosphamide (Cytoxan), and methotrexate. How they work is quite another story.

It's possible that you've heard of these medications not in

connection with organ transplants, but in relation to malignant disease. Yes, they *are* so used (although SLE is *not* such a condition). They are being used in all three of these kinds of problems because of a particular effect that they have: they interfere, somehow, with cell proliferation, as well as with the production of antibodies. In cancer—which consists essentially of such intrusive proliferation—they thus head to the heart of the problem. It should be noted that they are effective in some types of cancer, but not in others; and we do not know that cancer, despite the single word denoting it, is in fact a single disease.

What is the connection? It's a tenuous one, and not yet fully understood. Such drugs tend to attack the most *rapidly* proliferating cells. Cells of cancerous growths generally multiply more rapidly than do normal cells. Bone marrow also normally manufactures blood cells—red cells and white cells—at a relatively high rate. Thus, such agents will have an effect there as well. (You might visualize such medications as entering the body and looking about for the most rapidly increasing kind of cells to attack.) White cells are prominent in the body's "immune" responses. Thus, the immunosuppressives, also called *cytotoxins* because they attack certain *cells* ("cyto" comes from *kytos,* Greek for "cell"), serve to diminish what may be, in SLE, an exaggerated immunological response.

Yes, these agents do behave somewhat indiscriminately; they may knock out the body's natural defenses against infection, as well. Three considerations obtain.

First, physicians will tend to prescribe such drugs quite carefully and typically only on a short-term basis—that is, not indefinitely. It is a sort of contest: try to get the medication to do what it is *supposed* to do, but don't let it "take over" and begin to destroy the body's defenses against infectious disease.

Second, the physician may decide upon a combination of two or more such drugs, perhaps with one of the corticosteroids. Both studies in experimental animals and controlled clinical studies in patients have suggested that sometimes—although not always—such combinations may be superior to a single drug. At this writing, such studies are still ongoing; rheumatologists are following them, and their results, with great interest. These drugs are still categorized as investigational medications. A physician should ethically inform you (in any case), *whatever* your condition and *whatever* the medications prescribed, what therapy you are receiving and why, and what it may be expected to accomplish; this holds true no matter what your medical situation.

Third, despite the foregoing comment, chiefly because there are not enough rheumatologists available, the time of the physicians who deal with the arthritic disorders is terribly limited. It is part of our purpose to supplement—*not*, we hasten to add, to *replace*—the information the individual physician gives his or her patient. As we noted earlier, these newer drugs are not ideal. They have drawbacks, and if you are taking one or more of them, it's important that you be aware of those drawbacks.

If you are taking one or more of the immunosuppressives, whether or not in combination with a cortisone type of medication, it's extremely important to be alert for inimical side effects. Such effects alert the physician that the drug has "gone over the line"—i.e., that it has begun to trigger unwanted and dangerous situations, and must be (at least temporarily) discontinued. Because individual reactions to the immunosuppressives may differ greatly, it's impossible to list potential "side effects," as we have done and will do for some other medications. What the SLE patient who is taking such drugs should watch

37

for is *any* untoward symptom whatever—i.e., anything that seems to be unusual, no matter how minor.

If you are taking any of these medications and you are a diabetic who takes insulin, you should, additionally, be on the alert for the increased possibility of an insulin reaction, which these medications seem sometimes to encourage. Methotrexate specifically dictates the avoidance of certain other substances that have been known on occasion to interact dangerously with this medication: alcohol, which can in such combination be speedily toxic to the liver; ordinary pain relievers, including aspirin, unless the physician has been consulted; tranquilizers or sedatives, again except on medical advice; and sulfa drugs.

Thus, it should be obvious that if one physician is being seen for an arthritic disorder and another for, say, an emotional problem or a respiratory infection, it is *vital* to alert each to what the other has prescribed.

Physicians are not mind readers. The ear, nose, and throat specialist consulted for a sinus infection will not know what other medication a patient may be taking *unless he or she is so informed,* whether by the patient or the referring physician; since the patient is the one who will suffer if someone else— whether doctor or assistant—neglects to pass on the information, it is a very good idea for the patient to assume that responsibility. At worst, information may be duplicated. At best, a lethal situation might be avoided.

Finally, it must be noted that cyclophosphamide, specifically, has been implicated in a number of cases of sterility, and that many of those cases have been irreversible.

Dermatomyositis

In many ways similar to SLE, dermatomyositis specifically attacks muscle, or skin and muscle, tissues; two thirds of adult victims, and even more children, do have skin involvement (in the absence of such involvement, the condition is sometimes termed *polymyositis*—"inflammation of many muscles").

Arthritis occurs in about half of all those who are afflicted by dermatomyositis, of whom 60 to 70 percent (estimates vary) are female. The age group attacked is fairly broad compared with SLE, although this particular disorder seems to appear most often in the forties, fifties, and sixties (bear in mind that dermatomyositis is quite rare compared with the other arthritic disorders—so that a far narrower sampling is available); but it has been known to occur in childhood.

As with SLE, the beginning symptoms of dermatomyositis often include a low fever; other initial signs may involve muscle tissues, skin, or both. There may also be some initial weight loss, as well as what physicians call "general malaise"—which most ordinary people describe as "I'm not feeling very well lately."

The muscular problem, initially, is usually weakness, possibly accompanied by a certain amount of pain; any muscles may be affected, but usually symptoms first appear in the muscles of, and connected with, the torso—the shoulders, hips, neck, and thighs. Muscles of the throat and chest may also be attacked eventually. Skin manifestations may take one or both of two forms. One: a pattern of scaly lesions similar to those of psoriasis, often occurring in the vicinity of joints such as the elbows or knees (unlike the cutaneous evidence of SLE—see page 27). More typical is a phenomenon often referred to as "heliotrope"

39

eyelids, a purplish discoloration of both the lids and the area surrounding the eyes; there is also often a puffiness—perhaps accompanied by a dusky-red discoloration—of the entire face, neck, and shoulders. (When these skin manifestations clear up, which they eventually do, there is often some residual mottling.)

In addition to these symptoms, which can of course suggest other problems, there are two laboratory tests that enable the physician to arrive at a diagnosis of dermatomyositis: a biopsy of muscle tissue and analysis of certain enzyme levels in the blood.

The cause(s) of dermatomyositis cannot, as you might imagine, be specified. With the limited research funds available, the least common arthritic disorders have suffered most. We do know that in some 10 to 50 percent of recorded cases of dermatomyositis in adults, a malignancy, frequently curable, has eventually turned up—and that the entire problem has disappeared upon the removal of the malignancy; among the sites of such malignancies have been the breast, lung, cervix, kidney, and gastrointestinal tract. (A question has been raised by researchers. Might the body, reacting against the invasive tumor —possibly caused by a virus or other infective organism—produce antibodies that also, as a sort of side effect, strike out against normal tissues? It should be noted that some researchers have turned up, in dermatomyositis, eccentrically behaving lymphocytes that seem to seek out and destroy muscle cells.)

We also know, purely statistically, that—again in adults—at least half of dermatomyositis victims (i.e., of those in whom the cause is unknown) are likely to survive the disease; but we must add that two out of five of those survivors, to date, have been moderately to severely disabled. In children, we have far less information, since the condition is both rare and relatively unlikely to strike this age group; often it is not diagnosed until fever and/or pain lead a child's parent to consult a physician, since prior muscular weakness can so easily go unnoticed. But so far as has been observed, the condition seems to be quite limited in youngsters, running about two years, and a combination of prompt diagnosis, treatment with corticosteroids, and physical therapy is generally successful.

In adults, the chief victims of dermatomyositis, therapy generally takes the same forms as for SLE—i.e., analgesics, steroids, immunosuppressive drugs, or combinations thereof. (Azathioprine in particular seems especially effective in creating apparently lasting remissions.) See pages 33–38.

Scleroderma (PSS)

The name of this condition—like dermatomyositis quite a rare one—derives, like a number of the medical terms we've defined, from Greek. The *derma* part, of course, means "skin." *Sclerosis* denotes a *hardening* process. Which seems to suggest "hard skin." Its alternate name, progressive systemic sclerosis (PSS), is at once more descriptive and more accurate; it does indeed affect the entire body, not merely the skin. Again, females lead males in recorded cases, apparently to a somewhat lesser degree than in the other two conditions we've discussed in this chapter; the ratio seems to be about three to two, possibly as high as two to one. The age range for PSS is broad, but there has been a concentration of recorded cases in the thirties, forties, and fifties.

Symptoms may or may not be initially visible. PSS—or its agent, whatever it may be (no connection with either infection or malignancy has been demonstrated)—may attack either skin or muscle tissue to start with. Usually, as with dermatomyositis, there are diffuse aches and pains initially, accompanied by fever. Other manifestations are extremely variable. If the skin is involved, the affected area may become shiny and waxy-looking and later harden, shrivel, and lighten. Mucous membranes may be similarly affected. If joints are involved, which they often are in PSS, the hands, for example, may swell and display symptoms similar to those of rheumatoid arthritis, although the discomfort is usually milder. An early sign might be muscular weakness—anywhere. Or localized edema (puffy swelling). Or gastrointestinal difficulties. Despite the multiplicity of possible symptoms, definitive diagnosis can be done via biopsies and other laboratory tests.

PSS is surely one of the most baffling entities in medicine. The one lead that has turned up is an unusually high incidence, in PSS patients, of chromosome peculiarities in certain of the blood's white cells—specifically, the lymphocytes. The reason is simply unknown (nor has any direct connection with the disease itself been proved); among the possibilities that have been suggested are hereditary abnormalities and/or damage perpetrated by a virus or other infectious agent. Such oddities have *not* emerged, by the way, in the other arthritic disorders.

We cannot be specific about the prognosis in PSS; far too little is known. Victims of it have been known to succumb within six months—or to survive to cope with the discomforts for twenty-five years. The use of cigarettes and/or alcohol seems statistically associated with a rapid worsening of the condition —although we cannot substantiate any direct connection. Severe hypertension (high blood pressure) is also associated with a poor prognosis. Specific medications, including the immunosuppressives found useful in SLE and dermatomyositis, have not been conclusively proved effective in PSS. Thus the search for a cause and concise therapy continues. Meanwhile, we must rely upon the general remedies for all of these painful problems: the analgesics, anti-inflammatory drugs, and, rarely, corticosteroids; they are discussed in Chapter 7.

FOUR

A Special Ill of Special People: Gout

In the last chapter, we explored three arthritic disorders that remain profound and often agonizing mysteries. Here, we encounter a horse of radically different hue. Gout is one of the most clearly understood of all the arthritic disorders and the most susceptible to rational control (though not *cure*; we'll shortly see why).

It wasn't always so. The Reverend Charles Lutwidge Dodgson, the nineteenth-century writer better known to several generations of adoring children and grownups as Lewis Carroll, wrote in *The Hunting of the Snark*, "There are certain things— as, a spider, a ghost, the income-tax, gout, an umbrella for three —that I hate." The Reverend Mr. Dodgson's coupling of gout with such fanciful threats as ghosts and the discomfort of trying to keep the rain off three heads with one umbrella was meant in jest; he well knew just how real, and how painful, the assault of gout could be.

Gout's hateful pangs have been known to man since ancient times; it was recognized and described as a distinct entity by Rufus of Ephesus in the first century A.D. Its very name, in fact, dates from those early days of medicine and the "humors" concept of illness we mentioned in Chapter 1. Because gout— or gouty arthritis as it is also, perhaps more accurately, known

45

now—often tends initially and predominantly to affect the joints of the big toe, it was theorized that whatever malevolent substances triggered the condition did so because they somehow *spilled down into* the toe; hence, the word's derivation from the Latin *gutta*, denoting a "flowing down" or "drop." Oddly enough, this concept does touch on the actual physical phenomena that take place in gout: there *is* in a sense a flowing of certain substances—but they are substances far more specific than vague "humors," and gravity has nothing to do with it.

Nor are some of the more recent popular rationalizations of gout any more accurate; they are perhaps even less so—although, again, there have been tenuous connections with the real explanation. Nineteenth-century ill feeling between the social classes prompted the lower ones, having observed that gout is more likely to afflict the more affluent, to postulate that it was a concomitant of luxurious life styles—and it was probably nice to imagine a vengeful deity punishing with cruel afflictions those who were fortunate enough to enjoy fine food and drink and other perquisites of the well-to-do provided by the sweat of lower-ranking brows.

That idea led, quite naturally, to a direct and ultimately classless attribution of gout to the eating of rich foods and careless imbibing of alcoholic beverages, particularly the latter. Those readers who are old enough may recall comic strips of the 1930s and '40s in which the protagonist was pictured paying the price for his reckless tippling by being prostrated by "the gout," a foot swathed in bandages propped up on a pillow, captive in his easy chair while his cronies trooped merrily by the window on their way to the local tavern. The victims were invariably in agony, the more so because of reminders by the more "righteous" characters that they had "brought upon themselves" this grievous state—which was depicted more as a comic inconvenience than a genuine ailment.

Arthritis Uratica

That is the technical medical term for what is commonly called gout, and it is most accurate of all. Gout is truly an arthritic condition, involving joint inflammation. And it results, specifically, from the deposit of crystalline substances called *urates* in the afflicted joints. Though alcohol may *exacerbate* the condition, it is certainly not a *cause*. Drinking without eating, in particular, can in fact trigger an acute gout attack—not because of the alcohol per se, but because metabolism is altered under such circumstances.

Though certain *foods* can trigger gout, they cannot be truly termed causes either. Gout is a metabolic disorder. Metabolism is a general word for those processes by which the body puts substances through various chemical changes (it derives from the Greek *metabole*, which means "change").

In gout, there is a metabolic defect that results in less than efficient handling of certain substances called *purines*, which are found predominantly in fatty meats and poultry (pork, duck, goose); in organ meats such as kidney, sweetbreads, and liver; in some game birds; and in certain fish and shellfish (clams, scallops, anchovies, etc.). When they are broken down by the body, one by-product of that process is uric acid; the uric acid goes into the bloodstream and eventually reaches the kidneys, where—in the normal course of events—excess quantities of it are filtered out to be excreted (it's *called* uric acid, in fact, because it is a major component of *urine*).

But in someone afflicted with gout, that process does *not* proceed normally, *either* because such an individual produces extraordinary amounts of uric acid, *or* because the kidneys fail to handle the excess quantities properly. The result is hyperuricemia, *hyper-* meaning "excess" and the suffix *-emia* (from the Greek *haima,* "blood") referring to the bloodstream—i.e., an excess of uric acid in the circulation. The acid, in combination with other elements, eventually forms solid, crystalline substances called urates, which the circulation proceeds to deposit at various points around the body. This process takes place especially in an acid environment; the solubility of these substances increases with alkalinity.

The depot points are primarily—though, as we shall see, not entirely—joints. We are not sure precisely why this is so, but recent research suggests that a particular protein substance, present throughout the body but especially highly concentrated in cartilage and in the synovium (the membrane lining a joint), constitutes a sort of "chemical welcome mat" for urate crystals. Theoretically, any joint is a likely candidate. Actually, certain joints tend to be singled out: the proximal joint of the big toe (the one closer to the foot)—affected initially in seven out of ten gout victims, eventually in 90 percent—and, less commonly, the fingers, instep, wrist, ankle, elbow, or knee. Rarely, a shoulder or that part of the spine in the region of the neck may be involved. Eventually, there may be urate deposits in the cartilage of the external ear, in the sheaths of the tendons and—if the condition is permitted to continue untreated—in the kidneys themselves (which, of course, is doubly critical because excretion of uric acid then becomes even less efficient).

Ultimately such deposits may form lumpy concentrations called *tophi* (that's a plural coming directly from Latin; the singular is *tophus*). In and around joints, tophi can create serious limitations of motion; in the kidney, they are called stones. They can also occur in quite unexpected sites, such as the eye—actually, just about anywhere in the body.

The foregoing describes, necessarily briefly and generally, the course of chronic, continuing gout. Gout is also manifested by periodic acute attacks—the episodes pictured in the aforementioned comic strips—that may be triggered by a variety of circumstances including injury (even minor injury, such as a stubbed toe), drinking of alcohol (especially, as previously noted, without eating), surgery, physical or emotional strain, and fatigue; these precipitating factors may vary from one individual to another. During an acute attack, the involved joint presents what is probably the most graphic picture of inflammation in all of medicine, with all the classic signs clearly in evidence (see page 6). There is swelling. There is a distinct sensation of heat. The skin of the affected area is red to purple, shiny in appearance. And there is severe pain; tenderness may be so acute that the slightest touch, or even a breath of air, proves agonizing.

At the onset, such attacks—a typical early attack lasts a day or two, several days at most—are usually few and far between. Later, attacks come more often, perhaps several times a year, and tend to last longer than earlier ones.

Who are the "special people" of our chapter title, the victims of gout? As we've pointed out, they are not necessarily the wealthy, or the wine-women-and-song crowd. Nor are they, as some have believed, necessarily the brilliant and the gifted—although it is true that many noted figures in history have been among the afflicted; Benjamin Franklin was perhaps the most famous gout victim, and others have included such diverse VIPs as Alexander the Great, British Prime Minister William Pitt, and poet John Milton. You will note that these people have one thing in common: they are all male.

Although we do not yet fully understand the precise biochemical mechanism in gout, we *do* know that it is a familial disorder. Unlike the situation that obtains with some of the other conditions discussed in this book, gout's origin is clear; the metabolic malfunction that creates it is an inherited genetic defect. And that heredity does have somehow to do with sex; of the roughly one million Americans known to be victims of gout, at *least* 950,000 are male. This would certainly seem to suggest a classic sex-linked recessive inheritance. But that pattern would not alone account for such overwhelming odds.

Possibly, as some believe, there is what has been termed a recessive-qualified, or recessive-plus, mode of inheritance: that is, *other* factors (perhaps genetic, perhaps not) may be operative as well. One such factor could well be the different hormonal make-up of the sexes: gout's onset is typically in the prime of life—the thirties, the forties—and virtually never begins as early as the teens; further, the women who *do* suffer from gout tend not to evidence the disease until after menopause. Thus some have postulated a protective role played by the female hormones. A few researchers have even theorized that the gene for gout is a *dominant* one, and that the hormones are *the* key factors in determining whether gouty arthritis develops or not. And other *acquired* factors—excess weight is one that is under strong suspicion—may well play a part in setting the scene for gout, given a hereditary susceptibility.

In late 1972, some interestingly relevant research findings were reported by Drs. Gerald Weissman of New York University and Giuseppe Rita of the University of Turin in Italy. Effects observed in laboratory experiments—involving only the isolated substances, not living human beings—indicated that only lysosomes (see pages 7–8) rich in cholesterol or in testos-

terone (a male sex hormone) are susceptible to the inflamma-
tion-triggering action of urate crystals. Further, it was determined that estrogen, a female sex hormone, lends resistance to
that action. Those observations may explain the higher incidence of gout in males, as well as in those who eat rich foods
(or who are inclined to be high blood-cholesterol producers—a
characteristic that is very probably *also* hereditary).

There is no way to prevent gout; the mode of inheritance,
whatever it may be, is beyond human control. Nor can gout
be cured, in the sense that an infection can be banished by an
antibiotic agent, or a fractured bone realigned so it may heal
and become whole once more. Happily, however, it *can* now be
controlled—so that someone who suffers from chronic gout
need never find himself in the pathetic predicament portrayed
in the cartoons.

Three-Way Therapy

Gout, again unlike some other arthritic disorders, can be
clearly differentiated from other similar-appearing conditions—
by a physician, not necessarily by the layman. Aside from
observed symptoms, the doctor can rely on blood tests that
demonstrate hyperuricemia, analysis of joint deposits, micro-
scopic examination of fluid drawn from the joint, sometimes
also X ray of the affected area. Once gout has been diagnosed,
treatment is instituted, with three objectives: to relieve the immediate inflammation; to prevent acute attacks in the future;
and to deal with the chronic situation—that is, to avoid continued deposit of urates and, if possible, to disperse present crystal concentrations and already-formed tophi in the joints and
elsewhere.

Physicians differ to some extent on whether certain diet controls should play a part, prominent or otherwise, in the treatment of gout. There's general agreement that high-purine foods should be shunned during an acute attack. Some feel that those strictures should be continued as a regular regimen; others believe that once a normal blood level has been achieved, medication alone (which must, as we'll see, be taken on a continuing basis, just as a diabetic takes insulin) is effective. A middle course seems reasonable: not necessarily regimenting the diet rigidly, but making some effort to curtail *provocative* factors, such as alcohol and high-purine foods—depending, of course, on the troublemakers for each individual.

Before we detail the nature of the unique medications that are now available for the treatment of gout, two other sometimes relevant factors should be noted. One is the presence of a weight problem. If a gout patient is obese to begin with, weight reduction does tend to have a beneficial effect: it lowers the degree of hyperuricemia; so in the long run, weight reduction will be one of the objectives. But the kind of diet needed for weight loss, conversely, tends—because it is typically relatively high in proteins—to *raise* the blood-urate levels.

No, it is not an insoluble dilemma. What the physician will generally advise is putting off the weight-loss program until an acute attack has passed; then, during the weight-reduction period, frequent blood tests will be done to keep a constant eye on the state of things, adjusting medication dosages if necessary in order to be sure of preventing acute attacks. Obviously—we suppose it's obvious, but we'll mention it anyway—such a weight-loss program is best undertaken with the advice and continuing supervision of the physician who is treating the gout.

The second complication is that sometimes, when treatment begins, tophi in the joints or tendons have already reached disabling proportions. It *is* possible to remove such formations surgically. But surgery itself can sometimes prove to be an at-tack-triggering factor, so that a physician is unlikely to advise it until chemical stabilization has been achieved and maintained for a while. By that time, the problem often resolves itself: most tophi tend to be resorbed once normal blood-urate levels have been reached and maintained. (The exception is the case in which kidney stones have already formed in such size or quantity that they are impairing kidney function or causing in-tractable pain; then, early surgery may be an unavoidable neces-sity.)

There are now a number of medications from which the physician can choose to treat the gout patient. They are, as previously noted, designed to deal with the acute inflamma-tion *and* to prevent further problems. With one exception, the medications used in an acute attack and those used for preven-tive treatment are totally different drugs.

The Acute Attack

Physicians are by no means insensitive to the exquisite agony of an acute attack of gout. They will hasten to call upon what-ever is available, with the aim of lessening the pain just as quickly as possible. Their first recourse, if there is a definite or at least highly probable diagnosis of gout, is *colchicine*.

Despite our castigation of folk remedies in general in Chap-ter 2, colchicine was not discovered in the modern chemistry lab, but in the field. Literally. It is an alkaloid derived from a plant botanically called *Colchicum autumnale*, a European herb known popularly as the meadow saffron or autumn crocus. The roots and seeds of the plant were being urged upon gout sufferers, so far as we can determine, as far back as the fifth or sixth century A.D., and some scholars believe the remedy may

53

even have been known in ancient Egypt. It was, however, a case of it-works-but-who-knows-why. Not until the early 1800s was the active ingredient, colchicine, isolated from the plant.

Colchicine (it is marketed under the generic name; there are no brand names) is now widely available in tablet form and also available as a solution for intravenous injection. What it *seems* to do is block the inflammatory reaction at the sites of urate crystal deposit. An injection, given at the first sign of trouble, can abort an attack in half an hour. If it's later, but still within the first two days, the oral drug may be tried. When the situation has persisted for forty-eight hours or more, colchicine is considerably less effective—and it is totally ineffective in most *other* types of arthritic inflammation, whatever the cause.

The other relevant characteristic of colchicine is that it is a superstrong cathartic, as many a gout victim will testify. Diarrhea is an invariable side effect. It usually doesn't occur with the first dose. The physician treating an acute attack of gout will continue the colchicine until there is relief of the discomfort or severe gastrointestinal upset evidences itself, whichever occurs first; this means the medication will be continued for twenty-four hours, usually considerably less. At that point, the dosage may be cut down considerably or even eliminated altogether. (In some individuals, there may be other side effects as well, though they are unlikely to occur with the short-term therapy used in an acute attack. A patient taking colchicine—as with any other drug—should be careful to follow the prescribed dosage, and to report any untoward reactions to the physician promptly.)

What if colchicine's side effects become unbearable, or the doctor feels the medication is proving ineffective or not working quickly enough, or the attack has been under way for forty-eight hours or more when the patient reaches the doctor? There are several effective anti-inflammatories available—not specific for gout, but usually effective against inflammation generally. ACTH, a pituitary hormone, may be given by injection along with the colchicine. Or, as a substitute for the colchicine, the physician may turn to one of the very potent anti-inflammatories such as indomethacin, phenylbutazone, or oxyphenbutazone (milder medications such as aspirin will have little or no effect and the corticosteroids, useful in some other arthritic disorders, are generally considered inadvisable in gout). These drugs, which are often employed in acute stages or "flare-ups" of other types of arthritis as well, are discussed in detail in Chapter 7.

Continuing to Cope

The various remedies for acute attack can cut short what might otherwise have been many days of agony. But they do not deal with the underlying problem: the metabolic disorder that afflicts the gout victim. That disorder, remember, is a chronic one and persists even when the inflammatory episode has ended. Which means that—until or unless a *cure* is discovered—the measures taken to deal with it must continue as well. Yes, for life. The physician, based upon precise assessment of the situation—extent of existing urate deposits, blood uric-acid levels, state of kidney function—now has four drugs from which to choose; they may be prescribed singly or in combination.

One is our old friend colchicine, which not only copes effectively with acute inflammation, but has the happy facility of helping to *prevent* attacks as well. It may totally eliminate the possibility of acute attacks—which may, as we noted earlier, be triggered by a variety of events—and it will at least render them less frequent. Usually the patient will be instructed to take the medication on a regular basis (the dosage is substantially lower than that used in an acute attack) and to add an extra dose if he feels an attack coming on; that fast action usually aborts the attack, since the earlier medication is taken, the more effective it is. Colchicine is most useful as prophylactic therapy in those gout patients who have had frequent acute attacks.

A second weapon in the antigout armamentarium is the type of drug called a *uricosuric*, of which there are two presently available: probenecid (Benemid) and sulfinpyrazone (Anturane). Uricosurics might also be called hypouricemics. What they do is create a higher level of uric acid in the urine (uricosuria) while lowering (hypo-) the level circulating in the bloodstream. In short, they increase the body's excretion of that troublemaking substance. Such a drug, too, is taken on a regular daily basis; generally the physician will check blood-urate levels periodically and may revise the dosage schedule—whether upward or downward—if that seems advisable. The object, of course, is to achieve and maintain a normal level, so precipitation and deposit of further crystals in the joints or elsewhere will be prevented. (As the blood level is lowered, body fluids can also begin to dissolve away existing deposits—although that effect is usually evident only after several weeks of therapy.) Probenecid is the less powerful of the two uricosurics, but it is also less likely to have toxic side effects (of which more shortly) and is therefore considered relatively safer over the long haul.

The uricosurics are especially helpful in those gout patients who have developed tophi in the joints, but have no kidney stones. They are contraindicated (considered inadvisable) in those who tend to excrete high levels of uric acid in the first

56

place, since sending additional quantities through the kidneys encourages the development of stones there.

The fourth, and newest, drug designed for continued coping with the underlying difficulty is allopurinol (Zyloprim), a substance quite different from the uricosurics. Allopurinol strikes at the heart of the problem by actually inhibiting the production of uric acid in the first place; it does this by blocking the action of a particular enzyme that plays a crucial role in uric-acid formation. Additionally, it is able to dissolve, to an extent, uric-acid stones that have formed in the kidney, so that it is especially helpful in cases involving kidney dysfunction or where the patient has been going through the extra agony of passing such stones; it is also an alternative to colchicine in those who have no specific kidney problems, but who tend to a higher-than-normal level of uric-acid excretion.

Problems and Precautions

All of these drugs, it should be borne in mind, are extremely potent; they *must* be, in order to accomplish their objective of modifying basic bodily processes. If you, or someone in your family, is taking one or more of them, some elementary precautions should be faithfully observed.

First, the prescribed dosage and frequency must be followed without deviation—in *any* direction. It should be left to the physician to change the regimen; if the drug does not seem to be doing its job, the doctor should judge whether the amount should be increased, or more time should be allowed ("if one is good, two is better" is *not* a good rule of thumb). Of course the medication *cannot* perform its assigned task if doses are omitted or forgotten (skipping a dose of allopurinol, in fact, can directly *precipitate* an attack).

Second, it is vital to be alert to side effects that may indicate some serious allergic or other idiosyncratic reaction. These are frequently unpredictable; the physician must depend upon the patient to report such reactions promptly—and again, the physician must be the judge of whether the reaction is a minor one (or even a manifestation of the disorder itself) or is to be considered serious enough that the drug in question should be reduced or even halted.

Since such reactions can be and often are highly individual, it is impossible for us to provide a "check list" of any and all eventualities; *any* unexpected symptom or other development means the doctor should be called without delay. In general, however, the following should be particularly noted and quickly reported. *Colchicine:* severe diarrhea; usually scanty or infrequent urination; any trace of blood in the urine; muscular weakness; any rash or itching; sore throat; sores in the mouth; numbness, pain, or weakness in hands or feet. *Probenecid:* headache; gastrointestinal problems, including nausea; loss of appetite; unusually frequent urination; dizziness; fever; sore gums; itching or rash. *Sulfinpyrazone:* reactions of the upper gastrointestinal tract (which can be minimized—but they should still be reported to your doctor—by taking the medication along with food or milk); rashes or itching; any discomfort or other untoward reaction in someone with a history of peptic ulcer; any urinary oddities whatever. (Note: this drug is chemically related to phenylbutazone, which is discussed in Chapter 7; hypersensitivity to one may apply to the other as well.) *Allopurinol:* unusual drowsiness; rashes or other skin eruptions; chills or fever; nausea, vomiting, diarrhea, or abdominal discomfort.

Third, these drugs are known to interact chemically with certain other medications that might be taken; such interactions may be extremely undesirable. This fact means that the gout patient should exercise due care in choosing and using over-the-counter remedies—and should, additionally, fully inform all the physicians concerned (i.e., if different doctors are being consulted for different problems) of all medications that are being taken.

Not all possible drug interactions are known; the following are some that are.

Colchicine. Be wary of depressants of any type (including sedatives, alcohol, tranquilizers, etc.), since colchicine can increase their effects. Avoid, if possible, use of sympathomimetics, drugs that have a decongestant effect and are present in many cold pills, nasal sprays, and the like (the most widely used are phenylephrine and phenylpropanolamine), but can also affect the nervous system generally; their effects are also increased by colchicine.

Probenecid. Don't take aspirin or drugs containing it, since they'll counteract the uricosuric action of the probenecid; headaches and the like can be alleviated with another mild over-the-counter analgesic such as acetaminophen (Tempra, Tylenol, Valadol, et al.). If antibiotic therapy is contemplated for another condition, the physician should be completely informed before one or another type is decided upon; probenecid inhibits the therapeutic effects of erythromycin by boosting fast excretion of this drug, while increasing the action of penicillins and cephaloridine by cutting down on their rate of excretion—though other major antibiotics, such as streptomycin and the tetracyclines, are apparently unaffected. Finally, if the gout sufferer is also a diabetic and is taking oral drugs (as opposed to insulin) for that condition, that should also be a topic for discussion with the doctor (or both doctors, if more than one is involved). With some—not all—of these drugs, there might occasionally be some interference with excretion of the drug; the effect has been noted primarily with acetohexamide (Dymelor).

Sulfinpyrazone. As with probenecid, aspirin and similar salicylates should be avoided, since they interfere with the sulfinpyrazone's therapeutic action. And there also seems to be interference with excretion of not only acetohexamide, but with other antidiabetic drugs of the sulfonylurea class as well: chlorpropamide (Diabinese), tolazamide (Tolinase), tolbutamide (Orinase); there does *not* seem to be any interaction with the other type of antidiabetic, phenformin (DBI, Meltrol). Sulfinpyrazone also enhances the effects of injected insulin, so that someone on a regular insulin regimen should be doubly alert to the possibility of insulin reaction (and might ask the doctor about the possibility of decreasing insulin dosage). There has also been some suggestion that sulfinpyrazone blocks, to an extent, the excretion of anticoagulants (such as warfarin or phenindione), thus boosting the blood level of such drugs; again, as with the other medications we've mentioned, the situation should be discussed with the physician(s) involved, who may want to adjust the dosage of the other drug or may feel that tests for the precise effects in the individual are desirable.

Allopurinol. Certain of the interactions are so well known that any physician will be aware of the possibilities; they involve some of the other drugs used for gout, as well as some diuretics, certain immunosuppressives—azathioprine (Imuran) in particular—acetohexamide, and anticoagulant drugs. One that patients should be aware of is the danger of combining this drug with iron supplements—which are, unfortunately, widely available as components of over-the-counter vitamin-and-mineral products. It so happens that overdoses of certain vitamins are possible—not merely for the gout victim, but for anyone—and, further, that a perfectly adequate amount of these nutritional constituents is readily available via ordinary foods, assuming there is no medically verified deficiency. But our concern is at this point quite specific. Allopurinol can increase absorption of iron, hence the level of iron in the liver, which can itself be toxic; such an iron "overload" can be especially dangerous in older men, involving not only the liver, but the heart, pancreas, and other organs as well. As a general rule, whether one is taking allopurinol or not, it is a good idea to resist the intensive promotional pleas to gobble extra pills; if one is attracted to that idea, one's doctor is the person who should make the decision.

Addenda: The Goutlike Mysteries

We've described, in this chapter, the usual mechanism, manifestations, and treatment of gout—or arthritis uratica. By and large, the why and wherefore are pretty well understood, at least in comparison with some of the other arthritic disorders. For the sake of completeness, though, we must add that there are curiously similar conditions that *aren't* so satisfactorily pinpointed.

One is hyperuricemia itself—i.e., the presence of abnormally high blood concentrates of uric acid. Hyperuricemia almost invariably figures in gout. Yet the converse is not necessarily true. As a matter of fact, only some 10 percent of those individuals with demonstrable hyperuricemia actually develop gouty arthritis. Why? We don't know.

A second is the fact that both hyperuricemia and gout associated with it *can*, it is increasingly evident, occur as a sort of "extra complication" of quite different basic disorders. (Physicians are inclined to refer to such a situation as "secondary gout.") Among those that have been documented are effects of certain medications, malfunctions of the thyroid gland, cardio-vascular problems, some kidney diseases, lead poisoning, and a few types of malignancies.

And then there is a mysterious condition, recognized only recently, called *pseudogout* (mainly for lack of a better term). Frequently this problem is unearthed when a presumed victim of classic gout fails to respond to colchicine in an acute attack. Further investigation may reveal that inflammation of the affected joint (often *not* a big toe, as is typical in gout, but some other joint, such as the knee) has arisen from the deposit there not of urate crystals, but of crystals of inorganic calcium salts —in particular one called calcium pyrophosphate—which tend to lodge in cartilage and other soft tissues of the joint. (Another name for this condition is *chondrocalcinosis*, the first part of the word signifying *cartilage*.) We know that this substance is normally involved in bone formation. How does the body produce it? Why is it sometimes deposited in joint tissues? Might the condition be familial? Why is it almost invariably a precursor of osteoarthritis? We don't know.

Further, just to deepen the mystery, there may be a *form* of pseudogout minus the established symptoms—i.e., a condition in which calcium pyrophosphate is deposited in the joint *fluids*, typically resulting in synovitis (inflammation of the enveloping membrane of the joint) but *not* in involvement of the cartilage and other tissues. This condition tends mainly to affect knees and wrists, and bears an uncanny resemblance to rheumatoid arthritis (from which it can be quickly differentiated by spotting of the telltale deposits).

We have learned a good deal about these metabolic disorders in recent years, but there is a great deal left to learn. "Let knowledge," urged Lord Tennyson, "grow from more to more." Amen.

FIVE

Aches That Await Us All: Osteoarthritis

We come, now, to the kind of arthritis most of us think of when the word "rheumatism" is mentioned. If you play word association with the latter, we'll venture you'll come up with a list that includes old, grandparent, stiff, cold, "creaky." We are willing to wager you will *not* instantly associate it with any of the following: young, family, athletic, accident, graceful. Yet the second group of words is just as legitimately associated with this condition as the first.

It may as well be stated right off that this ailment is named quite inaccurately. Based upon the definitions in Chapter 1, osteoarthritis, because "osteo" refers to bone, would seem to indicate an inflammation of a joint, intimately involving the bone. Bone is involved, and so is the joint; but inflammation basically is not. *Osteoarthrosis,* i.e., a joint condition involving bone—a term current in Great Britain—would be more accurate. Even more specific is the sometimes applied but more lengthy phrase "degenerative joint disease"—because that's really what it is. Now that we have made that clear, we'll continue to refer to our topic as osteoarthritis, simply because that's the way it's generally known in the United States. Or, for short, OA. An essentially *non*inflammatory degenerative disease involving the joints.

And to satisfy your curiosity about those apparently out-of-the-blue words listed in the first paragraph, the condition has been known to afflict people in their twenties, persons (of any age, but particularly females in their forties) whose mothers evidenced the same problem, football players, people who suffered injuries at some time in the past, and ballet dancers. And we might add, miners, construction workers, good runners, poor runners, and people who are overweight.

If you surmise that might include everyone, or almost everyone, you're quite right.

There are, probably, people who will never have OA; they are, however, rare. We hasten to concede that there are many people who will not suffer substantially from it. But ninety-seven out of one hundred people will have it, to one degree or another, if they live long enough. "Long enough" may mean until the age of twenty-three—or the age of ninety-three. It all depends. But enough of the mystery. Just what *is* this malady that awaits virtually all of us?

A Wearing Away

Within all of our movable joints, intervening between bone and bone, cushioning and easing the movement of the joint, is a smooth, strong, elastic, self-lubricating, fibrous substance called *cartilage*. In OA, the cartilage in the affected joint very gradually softens, loses its elasticity, and begins to fray; as the process continues, pits, cracks, and fissures develop. These changes can be clearly seen if the tissue involved is examined under a device called a scanning electron microscope. Normal cartilage is a nice, smooth-looking substance with neatly aligned parallel bundles of fibers. The fibers of osteoarthritic cartilage are seen as twisted, roughly helical curlicues, with yawning gaps between them; in severe degeneration, they are totally disorganized and fragmented. Ultimately, if the condition progresses further (it may not), the cartilage disintegrates completely.

Meanwhile, as that cushion and easer of motion wears away, other parts of the joint are affected. The bone ends tend to thicken, as well as to develop "spurs" or bony outgrowths at the joint margin; these are called osteophytes—the last part of the word derived from the Greek *phyton*, "plant" (or, loosely, "growing thing"), the whole simply meaning "bony growth." Surrounding ligaments—connective bands between various joint structures—are also inclined to thicken somewhat, while adjacent muscles may weaken to a degree or contract unnaturally (i.e., become "tense" or "stiff").

No one knows precisely how or why this situation occurs, because no one knows, at this point, precisely how cartilage is built up in the first place, let alone how it breaks down. (In 1973, at a medical meeting of the Arthritis Foundation, Drs. Marcel Nimni and Kalindi Deshmukh of the University of Southern California Medical Center in Los Angeles reported finding distinct abnormalities of chemical structure in collagen obtained from the cartilage of osteoarthritic joints. Whether these abnormalities represent a *cause* of cartilage degeneration or, on the other hand, reflect a *result* of that degeneration is not yet clear.) But we do know quite a bit about some *other* facets of OA. We know—because it is so prevalent, and there has been so much opportunity to gather data over the years—whom it is likely to affect, when in life the degenerative process is likely to start, and which joints are most likely to be affected.

That last is an extremely important point. Unlike any other condition discussed in this book, OA *is not a systemic disorder.* It does not manifest itself in generalized symptoms such as fever or chemical abnormalities detectable in the bloodstream. Nor will it go galloping about the body from one joint to another. Its impact is strictly circumscribed, limited to the particular joint or joints it attacks. If, in other words, an individual suffers from OA in more than one part of the body, it's coincidence rather than manifestation of a systemic illness.

Whom OA is likely to strike is something we've already mentioned: almost everyone. The process—the degeneration of cartilage in joints that will ultimately be affected—starts (aside from special circumstances we'll mention shortly) quite early; estimates range from the early twenties to the thirties. According to the latest census figures, 54 percent of the U.S. population is twenty-five years of age or older; we may assume that in nine out of ten, OA has to some degree begun.

Not that awareness of the condition is likely to take place at those ages; those who are aware of the osteoarthritic process at twenty-five are extemely rare—although, as we'll see, not nonexistent. Awareness comes with symptoms and, if they are sufficiently severe, with doctor visits and precise diagnosis. The National Center for Health Statistics, an arm of the U. S. Department of Health, Education, and Welfare, estimates that OA is evident in 54 percent of American men between the ages of forty-five and sixty-four, in 57.5 percent of women in the same age group; in those aged sixty-five to seventy-nine, the figures are 77 percent for men, 86 percent for women. OA accounts for about 55 percent of all cases of severe arthritic disorders in the United States, afflicting one in twenty Americans; as we achieve longer life, that is likely to increase.

You'll note that the figures are slightly higher for women—not radically so, as with some of the other arthritic disorders, but nonetheless OA is clearly more prevalent among females. We are not quite sure whether OA in general strikes more women than men. If it does, the differences are probably slight and relatable to the slight predominance of females in our general population, or the statistics are perhaps due to women's greater willingness to seek medical care. There is, however, a *type* of OA that is unquestionably female oriented, and likely influences the overall statistics.

Handed Down

This particular type of OA is, like gout, hereditary, but with sex preference reversed. It probably should have a particular name, but it doesn't; it's classified in OA because the physical picture is the same as that in any other kind of OA—except for the site, the consistent time of onset of symptoms, and the hereditary pattern. This particular type strikes, quite specifically, the fingers (rarely, the toes). Just for purposes of avoiding lengthy phrases for the next couple of paragraphs, we're going to coin a term for this condition. The bones of the fingers are, anatomically, the *phalanges* (that word can also be applied to the toes). So we shall call this special condition phalangeal osteoarthritis: POA.

The typical victim of POA is a woman—the ratio is ten to one—in her forties (give or take a few years) whose mother evidenced the same condition. She will likely first notice a thickening of particular joints of her fingers, often especially the index and third fingers; the joints involved are, almost always, the distal (farthest from the torso) interphalangeal (between bones of the fingers) joints—or, as they're often called for short, the DIP joints. These thickenings, which are of course evidence of osteophyte formation, are termed, in deference to the eighteenth-century British physician who first singled them out as a characteristic of POA, Heberden's nodes. Sometimes the second, or proximal (PIP), joints display the same signs; thickenings there are often referred to as Bouchard's nodes, after the nineteenth-century Frenchman who pointed *them* out (the separate name is a little silly, and probably unfair to Dr. Heberden, since the phenomenon is identical). About 20 percent of those with POA have both types; Bouchard's nodes very rarely occur alone.

Usually POA, at least at the onset and often later as well, is relatively painless. Occasionally, there is some discomfort. But by and large, and in clear contrast to the OA situation in general, the osteophytic factor predominates. Further setting POA apart is the fact that the site is consistent and completely *un*related to prior use or abuse of the joints involved. Which brings us to the broader, the near-universal, phenomenon.

But before we go on to that, one final, vital warning. The reader who has the symptoms we have described, but has not seen a doctor, should not leap to diagnostic conclusions. Apparent "Heberden's nodes" have been known to appear—for unknown reasons—in association with a number of serious systemic disorders, including heart disease, ulcerative colitis, and various malignancies. Any symptoms, no matter how innocuous they may seem, should be checked out by a physician.

Historic Hints

Although OA is often spoken of as a general "wear and tear" disease, implying that all of us, and all of our joints, are equally susceptible—that isn't true. Nor is the mere fact of growing older, as some have supposed, the key factor; again, if that were so, we'd all expect eventually to be afflicted with OA in all of the joints of our bodies.

In point of fact, OA occurs selectively. As the Arthritis

Foundation phrases it, "A perfectly functioning joint is least prone to OA; a joint which operates imperfectly, for whatever reason, is most susceptible." It is the joint with a history of special stress that is the likely candidate. For most of us, the stress is the stress of everyday living, and OA will develop only after that stress has persisted for some time; hence, symptoms will not appear until the late thirties at the earliest, more commonly the forties or fifties or even later. The more severe the stress, the faster cartilage breakdown will take place, and the earlier OA is likely to set in.

What are these stresses that can lead to imperfect function, thence to OA? There are a number of them.

One is a congenital structural defect. A joint that is malformed, so that it has never functioned quite properly, will be under constant stress; in such a joint, OA is likely to occur relatively early in life.

Another is injury. Dislocation, fracture, sprain, even severe bruising will leave a joint in less than optimum condition; the more disruptive the injury, the greater the likelihood of subsequent OA. (It should be noted, too, that in instances of injury, an *un*injured joint may suffer as well; thus if a knee, for example, is injured—hence, "favored"—the hip and ankle will be under some compensatory stress.)

A third is prior disease that has afflicted the joint—another form of arthritis earlier in life, for example, or a systemic infection that involved the joint, or a childhood bout with a disorder such as Legg-Perthes Disease (page 92)—especially if it was not promptly and properly treated.

A fourth sort of stress might be anything that subjects a joint to unusual strain, that in a sense "overworks" it. Joints thus looming large as potential OA targets would include the weight-bearing joints, primarily hips and knees, of the obese;

the knees of certain athletes; the ankles and toes of dancers; the fingers of bowlers; the fingers of wrestlers (which are frequently broken); the spinal joints of laborers who continually bend over to lift heavy loads; joints of those whose poor posture results in uneven weight distribution, placing undue strain on one joint or another and resulting in center-of-gravity displacement that may especially dispose to OA of one or both hip joints. (In actual incidence, not all joints of the body seem equally susceptible—given comparable stresses—to OA. Knees, hips, and—less commonly—certain sections of the spine are involved far more often than, say, ankles or elbows. We don't know why this is so, but researchers are studying the mechanisms of the various joints for possible clues.)

These suppositions have been borne out both by clinical observation and by specific investigations.

In 1971, for instance, a group of Canadian football players— fifty-nine of them—were thoroughly examined and X-rayed, and the results compared with identical studies of fifty-nine "controls," young men of the same average age (twenty-three) who were *not* professional athletes. Some signs of OA were found in 4 percent of the latter group. But *all* the football players evidenced signs of OA, and in seven out of ten, the condition had progressed to a stage advanced enough to be medically termed severe. The afflicted joints were primarily knees and ankles, and the worst cases were found in linemen—who play in a crouch position, their knees and ankles continuously flexed.

A European study reported in 1972 gave added substance to the probable role of such flexing. That report cited an unusual incidence of OA of the knees in auto mechanics and others who habitually work in a squatting position. And it made an additional point that relates to something we mentioned earlier—the part played by the structure of the individual joint.

It is possible that the range of presumably normal joint structure should be more fully explored. Some long looks *have* been taken at *knees*. It is now known that there are a number of variations—relating both to the shape of the kneecap and to its position within the joint, especially in relation to the thigh bone—among apparently perfectly normal knees. Perhaps because of these structural differences, the cartilage in some knees will be more greatly stressed by a particular action or position than that in others. That would explain why, although many athletes—football and hockey players in particular—eventually are OA victims, some are not. And of course not *all* those who are obese, or have experienced joint injuries, inevitably suffer OA in the "expected" sites; again, inherent structural factors may make the difference.

Display and Detection

Initially, there may be no subjective symptoms at all; there have been cases in which doctors have discovered clear evidence of OA on an X ray taken for some other purpose—much to the surprise of the patient, who had experienced no discomfort whatever. Usually, however, subjective symptoms of OA antedate signs that the physician can detect objectively.

OA typically first shows itself by a mildly achy feeling in and around the joint, especially when it has been in use. That discomfort isn't felt principally by the cartilage or bones, since they contain few nerve endings, but by muscles and other surrounding tissues. In fact, curiously, the pain or discomfort may not be felt in the area of the joint itself at all; because of reflexive muscular responses, it may be what physicians call *referred* to a nearby area. This applies particularly to OA of the hip, of the cervical (neck area) spine, and of the lumbar spine (the lower back); in other joints, discomfort *is* usually localized. The ache of OA of the hip may be referred to the groin, buttocks, thigh, or back of the knee; that of the cervical spine, to the shoulders and arms; that of the lumbar spine, to the legs.*

The second common symptom is stiffness: the joint does not move easily and comfortably. This lack of flexibility is especially noticeable after the joint has been rested for a while—on getting out of bed in the morning, for instance, or, with OA of the hip or knee, after prolonged sitting in one position; with continued motion of the joint, it tends to "loosen up," and the stiffness dissipates fairly quickly.

These two characteristics, along with the usual lack of inflammation, help to distinguish OA from rheumatoid arthritis, a quite different disorder we'll be talking about in the next chapter. In OA, increased motion through the day means increased pain, which subsides with rest—while the pain of RA, which is also typically more intense rather than achy, does *not* disappear with rest, and is commonly worst in the morning.

A third interesting symptom that often—though not always—occurs in OA of the knee or hip is a sensation that patients describe variously as "grating" or "roughness" when the joint is moved. In an advanced case, this "grating" can sometimes actually be felt, and heard as a faint "crackling," by the physician; it's called *crepitus* (from the Latin *crepo*, "rattle"), and it's similar to the sound you can hear when you rub a strand of hair, held very close to your ear, between your fingers. Both sound and sensation result, of course, from the rasp of bone against bone as the cartilage in the joint deteriorates.

How bad is OA likely to become?

By and large, when small joints are involved, the pain is

* OA of the spine is sometimes called spondylosis, from the Greek *spondylos*, "vertebra"—i.e., "spine disorder."

seldom intense; nor does the situation usually become markedly worse as time goes by. The exception to these reassurances is OA of the hip, in which the pain can become intense, there can be continuing damage, and deformity and severe limitation of motion can eventually result. We'll come shortly to remedies, both for such complications and for the ordinary garden-variety discomforts. First, a word about diagnosis.

Despite the fairly clear pattern we've described, OA can easily be mistaken for other conditions—and vice versa. There are many other things that can cause very similar symptoms, that require radically different treatment, and must be ruled out before a patient can be told that a stiff knee or aching back is "just" OA. And OA, which we've declared unequivocally is a *non*inflammatory disorder, can sometimes be accompanied by a certain amount of inflammation, complete with all the classic signs including redness, swelling, and a sensation of warmth—not due to the OA itself, but to irritation and inflammation, by bits of disintegrating cartilage, of the synovial membrane enveloping the joint. How does the doctor tell the difference?

There are a number of techniques at the physician's command. Obviously, a thorough physical examination, an accurate description of symptoms, and a history of prior joint stress are basic. The presence of fever, nondeliberate weight loss, or other generalized symptoms will lead the doctor to look in other directions, since OA causes none of these; as will a pattern of ostensibly typical OA symptoms in a comparatively young person who is not an athlete and has no history of either trauma or congenital defect affecting the involved joint.

Blood tests can at least tentatively screen out the other arthritic disorders. In all of them, there are certain detectable abnormal elements or qualities present in a significant percentage of patients; no such abnormalities are present in OA. Such tests will certainly be performed if inflammation is present (an inflamed knee, for example, can appear at first to be gout or pseudogout).

Joint fluid may be withdrawn for analysis, if the possibility of some other condition is suspected. One such possibility is infection within the joint, and analysis will then reveal the presence of bacteria; among the agents that are known to cause conditions that can at first seem much like OA are gonococcus, pneumococcus, staphylococcus, and streptococcus.

Finally, there is the vital bottom line: X ray. On the X-ray film, the physician can clearly see the characteristic bony spurs, the osteophytes, that confirm the suspicion of OA; even prior to osteophyte formation, X ray can reveal the narrowed space between the bone ends, where the cartilage is degenerating. Sometimes, it's true, subjective symptoms can appear very early in the process, before the condition shows up on X rays. But in that case—assuming thorough tests have eliminated all other possibilities—the doctor's diagnosis of OA will be tentative and, since X-ray-able signs *will* appear sooner or later in OA, follow-up films will probably be suggested. No diagnosis of OA can be conclusively verified without positive X-ray evidence.

Treatment

One of the most heartening advances in medicine in recent years—heartening both to rheumatologists and to those of their patients who have been painfully disabled by OA and other disorders—has taken place in the field of orthopedic surgery. As we noted earlier, such disability can sometimes occur in OA of the hip.

Now, it is possible for surgeons, using wondrously engineered devices of plastic and metal, to *completely replace* an inoperative hip joint and restore mobility; these operations have been performed successfully on patients as old as eighty. Such surgery, unknown a few short years ago, is now virtually routine in major hospitals and medical centers; it has been estimated that as many as twenty thousand total-hip-replacement operations were performed in 1972. In 1971, clinical trials of similar procedures for disabled knees (more of a problem in other disorders, particularly rheumatoid arthritis, than in OA) began; by mid-1972, more than one hundred of those procedures had been performed, with excellent results.

The joint-replacement operation is called *arthroplasty*, the second part of the word from the Greek *plastos*, meaning "formed" or "shaped"—i.e., joint remolding.

Arthroplasty is of course reserved for cases of extreme disability, which are fairly uncommon in OA. How are less severe cases treated? You will recall that the osteoarthritic process involves loss of cartilage. Cartilage, once lost, can't be regrown. A possibility that has occurred to researchers is that of a substance—something thick, fluid, and resilient—that might be injected into the joint, something that would flow smoothly around the bone ends, cushion them, banish discomfort, and restore flexibility. That idea is being pursued, and some feel that such treatment may be available within the decade. But finding a substance that is not only workable but safe—that will not trigger an even more critical problem, as foreign substances introduced into the body are frequently wont to do—will not be an easy task.

Meanwhile, the aim of treatment is twofold: to relieve pain and to keep the affected joint as mobile as possible. So far as medications go, aspirin and other simple analgesics, the kind available in any drugstore without prescription, are often enough

75

to do the trick—although the most effective dosage and schedule for taking them may not be the same as that advised on the label (the regimen should be discussed with the doctor). In infrequent episodes of acute pain, the physician may recommend more potent prescription drugs such as indomethacin or phenylbutazone. The corticosteroid hormones aren't used systemically in OA, but may occasionally be injected directly into the joint to relieve extreme pain. None of these drugs is limited to use in OA; all are discussed in detail in Chapter 7.

Another way in which the physician can help, in some instances, is with physical therapy. The OA patient should discuss with his or her doctor the possible advantage of a program of special exercises to flex the involved joint and, if necessary, to correct postural irregularities.

But in OA, perhaps more than in any of the other arthritic disorders, much of the care and treatment is in the patient's own hands. And there are a number of things the sufferer from OA can do.

One is certainly protecting the involved joint(s) from additional stress or strain that is sure to speed the disease process as well as perpetuate discomfort. A firm step in that direction, when the lower back, the hip, or any leg joint is involved, is to relieve some of the burden the joint is carrying: i.e., to lose excess poundage, get down to proper weight (to be determined by the doctor, not by ads or other sources), and stay there.

Whatever seems to aggravate the problem is obviously best avoided. Sometimes that's not as simple as it sounds, especially if one's life style must be altered; habits are often not easily changed. But realism dictates, for example, that favorite sports that make the situation worse be abandoned; sometimes a less strenuous activity can be substituted—billiards instead of bowling, for example, or golf rather than tennis. A housewife who has OA of the hip will often find that climbing stairs is a cause of exacerbation; reorganizing work schedules to cut such trips to a bare minimum will help. For anyone with OA, simple avoidance of general fatigue has a salutary effect.

Associated foot problems can also add to the strain of OA when a hip or knee is involved. Comfortable, well-fitted shoes are thus a paramount consideration—and styles that tend to throw the body out of line, such as extremely high heels, should be shunned. Existing problems that interfere with easy walking—painful calluses, corns, bunions—should be discussed with the physician, who may recommend treatment by a podiatrist (foot specialist).

Finally, extreme cold seems to make the pain of OA a good deal worse. Conversely, heat often provides welcome relief from persistent aches, basically by relaxing the tense muscles surrounding the affected joint; we delve into this topic in further detail in Chapter 8.

SIX

The Mystery Cripplers:
Rheumatoid Arthritis and Kin

The group of arthritic disorders comprised of rheumatoid arthritis, the very closely related psoriatic arthritis, and ankylosing spondylitis are of more concern—to physicians and patients alike—than any of the others, for it is these that are potential perpetrators of the most severely crippling and debilitating deformities. Together they afflict at least six million, and perhaps as many as ten million, Americans—chiefly in the prime of life, sometimes as early as the teens and even childhood.

The Arthritis Foundation estimates that some five million suffer from rheumatoid arthritis—but since a number of authorities feel that perhaps 20 to 40 percent of rheumatoid arthritis victims have relatively mild disease and never consult a doctor, the actual figure may be over six million and perhaps as high as eight million three hundred thousand. Approximately 5 percent of them are children. The baffling skin condition called psoriasis afflicts 2 to 5 percent of our population at one time or another; one in ten cases is accompanied by symptoms that are for all intents and purposes indistinguishable from those of rheumatoid arthritis. Ankylosing spondylitis, a distinct disorder affecting the back, claims at least half a million victims.

These quite serious ills pose particularly frustrating problems

79

in part because they are often extremely painful and can deform and disable, and because their courses are so unpredictable. Moreover, very little is known as yet about their causes; hence, even less about possible curative measures, except as symptoms and effects can be countered as they occur—which does not, of course, dispel the underlying disease. In this chapter, we summarize the known facts about each.

Rheumatoid Arthritis (RA)

What we say here applies, except as specified otherwise, to psoriatic arthritis as well; juvenile rheumatoid arthritis, which often presents quite a different picture, is discussed separately (see page 90).

RA primarily strikes young adults; at least three out of four are women, and four out of five are under the age of forty. The onset is generally gradual: there is usually swelling, a moderate degree of pain, and slight tenderness, typically starting in one or two small joints such as those of the fingers, wrists, or feet. Possibly there may be accompanying weakness, general fatigue, and stiffness when getting up in the morning (generalized, but worst in the involved joint or joints); sometimes there are also other symptoms, including loss of weight and appetite and, occasionally, fever. As the disease progresses, other joints such as the knees and/or hips may become involved.

It is the destruction caused by the inflammatory process in the joints, coupled with muscular reaction to pain, that can cause the severe deformity that sometimes occurs—particularly if treatment is not instituted early (the Arthritis Foundation has noted that, unfortunately, the average RA victim waits for three or four years before seeking treatment—resulting in a tragic amount of unnecessary crippling). Inflammation results in swelling of the synovial membrane that lines the joint, releasing agents that invade and eat away the cartilage that keeps the joint mobile. Meanwhile, spasm of surrounding muscles that has occurred as a reflex reaction to the pain has often pulled the joint out of line.

But as we have said, that result can in most cases be prevented—if the victim gets to the doctor in time. While RA presents a rather vague set of symptoms at first, there are clues that will lead the knowledgeable physician at least to suspect it. All that *can* emerge in early stages is suspicion, but that is sufficient to eliminate certain diagnoses and to put the condition—whether RA or some other disorder—under continuing, and crucial, observation.

Any one of the symptoms we have mentioned will lead the doctor to consider the possibility of RA. Certainly the physician will take a complete history and make a thorough physical examination. Aside from obvious swelling and inflammation, he or she will look for subcutaneous nodules that sometimes appear in (a minority of) RA patients after about a year. Beyond that, there are three laboratory tests that can be helpful, two of them at even the earliest stage of RA.

One is a blood value called the erythrocyte sedimentation rate (ESR), or "sed rate," as medical personnel generally refer to it; it is typically elevated in RA and some other rheumatic disorders. A normal ESR will in most instances exclude RA (in 10 to 15 percent of RA cases, the elevation does not occur). Another is the finding of a slight anemia, which is very characteristic of RA. The third is something called a latex fixation test, which can turn up a blood element termed a *rheumatoid factor*. It should be noted that (1) that factor is rarely present during the first year of RA; (2) it is present, later, not in all RA patients, but only in about 75 percent;

(3) it is not found in psoriatic arthritis; (4) it shows up, paradoxically, in many people who have no joint disease whatever. We do not know what the latter may mean. At this point we might inject some comment on:

The Cause. No one knows the full story. No familial factor has been demonstrated. RA occurs in all races and all climates; contrary to popular belief, low temperatures and dampness do not cause it (statistically, Eskimos have less RA than inhabitants of warmer, sunnier climes), although, as we shall note, climatic changes may affect its course.

Three major theories and one minor one prevail at this writing. One is a slow-virus mechanism (see pages 29–30). A second is an as yet unfathomed type of autoimmune reaction (again, a possibility in other ills as well; see pages 7–8). The third is a combination of the first two, a situation in which a virus (or viruses) may be involved and may trigger, essentially, an as yet ill-understood "allergic" reaction. Some—a minority—feel that RA should be classed with the metabolic diseases (such as diabetes) and will ultimately reveal an enzymatic or other clearly hereditary defect. The last is highly unlikely, unless what is involved is a hitherto unknown factor that plays a part in reaction to challenge—specifically, it would seem at this point, viral challenge. It is also quite possible that a *variety* of infectious agents can trigger the condition we now characterize as a single entity.

As in SLE, there have been investigations into the possible actions of myxoviruses, a particular class of viruses larger than the ordinary, run-of-the-mill type but smaller than bacteria. Such viruses have been isolated from RA patients, particularly a type similar to that which causes viral pneumonia. In one study, an extended course of tetracycline therapy was administered to such patients (some types of viral pneumonia are treatable with that therapy), but with no observable effects. It must be recalled, however, that in RA the viral invasion (assuming there is a viral invasion) may have taken place much earlier, and RA may in effect represent a "delayed reaction." In the intervening time, the virus might have been considerably strengthened (viruses are by nature parasitic and "feed" off their hosts). On the other hand, it must also be recorded that viral substances isolated from RA patients have *not* triggered RA—or, for that matter, *any* inimical reaction—in other, healthy subjects.

One final sidelight. There is a disease found in pigs, characterized chiefly by fever at the outset, which can be fatal. Those animals that recover from the acute phase of the illness thereafter suffer from a chronic arthritis that very much resembles RA in humans. During the first few months of the chronic illness, a specific bacterium, *Erysipelothrix insidiosa*, can be isolated from the sick animals; but later, though the arthritis continues, the bacteria seem to vanish into thin air and cannot be found in the pigs' arthritic joints or anywhere else! Researchers are continuing to study this phenomenon, since discovery of the presumed "hiding place" of the mischief-making bacteria in the pigs may well provide relevant clues to RA in people. (Some researchers—notably prominent scientists in the U.S.S.R., but including physicians here and elsewhere as well—are already convinced that in up to 75 percent of RA cases, onset of the arthritis is preceded by a bacterial infection, frequently strep and often involving the throat, with an interval of ten to fifteen days between the two events.)

Medication. Rheumatoid arthritis is perhaps the most individual disease there is. Unlike, say, osteoarthritis, it goes through spontaneous periods of activity and remission—and what causes (or seems to cause) a flare-up can vary considerably from one victim to another. The flare-ups can occur frequently or very infrequently; they may be mildly annoying or severely incapacitating. They appear to be triggered by factors as disparate as fatigue, abrupt changes in temperature or barometric pressure, and stressful emotional situations—again, peculiar to the individual. Often we find that RA improves during pregnancy, and may become considerably worse immediately after the baby is born; sometimes, in fact, it appears then for the first time.

The aim of therapy is essentially threefold: to relieve pain, to reduce inflammation, and to prevent crippling deformity. As you might imagine, it is unlikely that the course of the illness in any two patients will follow precisely the same pattern. Thus, the prescription of remedies will be highly individual. It is very much a trial-and-error situation, and the physician actually depends a great deal on the patient, both to cooperate in following the prescribed regimen and to report the results.

The RA patient should be aware that part of the problem is the coming-and-going nature of the arthritis. Did the medication work, or was there going to be a remission anyway? Your doctor is of course familiar with the relative efficacy of various drugs, and he or she can also judge their effectiveness in objective terms, by examination, periodic joint measurement, functional challenges, and other means; but your doctor also depends on you to report your feelings.

What medications are useful in rheumatoid arthritis?

Certainly the basic analgesics and anti-inflammatory drugs: the over-the-counter pain relievers, the more potent analgesics and anti-inflammatories in periods of acute pain. These, because they apply to almost all types of arthritis, are discussed in Chapter 7. What we might add here is that you may be asked to take such a drug on a regular basis even when you

84

are totally without pain or discomfort; this is a prophylactic, or preventive, measure, and it is important that the prescribed regimen be followed—since it can often prevent a dreadfully painful episode. The corticosteroids, as well, are used in RA; they are also discussed in detail in Chapter 7.

Some of the medications mentioned in Chapter 3 have been fairly extensively used for RA in the past. The antimalarial drugs (pages 33–34), because of their high potential for precipitating toxic reactions, are being used less and less—and in psoriatic arthritis, they are specifically contraindicated. The immunosuppressives (pages 35–38), which have proved useful in systemic lupus erythematosus and dermatomyositis, are now used very, very rarely in RA, since exhaustive studies have established that the dosages necessary often are highly toxic, so that these drugs are employed only when there has been no response to safer therapy; the exception is methotrexate, which has often proved beneficial in psoriasis.

There is, however, one particular type of drug that has been found beneficial *only* in rheumatoid arthritis: gold. The treatment is sometimes called aurotherapy, more often chrysotherapy (from the Latin and Greek words for gold, respectively *aurum* and *chrysos*). No, no connection with the copper bracelets and similar superstitions we dismissed in Chapter 2. In chrysotherapy, the gold is not worn on the wrist, but injected into the body. And it is not the familiar form of gold that is used, but one of a specific group of soluble salts, either gold sodium thiomalate (Myochrysine), gold sodium thiosulfate, or gold thioglucose (Solganal).

Gold salts were first tried for RA in the late 1920s. Over the next several decades, with much experimentation in dosages and courses of therapy, it became apparent to physicians and patients alike that chrysotherapy does work. Not until 1971, however, were results of a significant double-blind study announced, results that confirmed the observations and instincts of countless clinicians. A double-blind study is one in which neither the patient nor the physician knows what drug is being administered—so there is no chance of "anticipating" results or judging effects other than impartially.

In this particular study, half the group of RA patients—all of whom had suffered from arthritis for less than five years—were given actual gold salts, while the other half of the participants were given an innocuous "placebo," a substance made up deliberately to look precisely like a solution of gold salts. The results were definitive. The arthritis continued on its inexorable course in those patients who received the placebo. But 77 percent of those who received the real medication experienced both subjective and objective improvement—and in 23 percent, there was an apparently lasting remission.

Gold salts, then, are obviously effective in early stages of RA (they cannot reverse existing deformities)—although it must be noted that no one knows precisely how and why they work. Should chrysotherapy be *the* treatment for *all* rheumatoid arthritis? No, because unfortunately it is far from ideal, for several reasons.

One reason is that, as demonstrated, it does not seem to work in all patients. Another is that there is a relatively high incidence of hypersensitivity (allergy) to the drug, roughly 20 percent; once such a reaction takes place with any potent medication, it must be discontinued.

The third and most crucial reason is that gold is a toxic substance; it has been known to cause chromosome damage in lymphocytes, leukopenia (a dangerous depletion in the body's circulating white cells), anemia, excretory abnormalities, and, rarely, nephrosis (a serious degenerative kidney disorder).

We hasten to add that these toxic and potentially fatal effects, if they are pinpointed, can generally be reversed by the administration of certain drugs—notably two chemicals called N-acetylcysteine and British antilewisite (also known as BAL or by its generic name, dimercaprol), which are specific antidotes for metal poisoning—and/or corticosteroids. With care, such effects can be prevented. But awareness on the part of both physician and patient is vital; there must be recognition of the risks and alertness to danger signals.

(Illustrative of the unpredictability of gold therapy was another study reported in 1971. Among a group of RA patients treated with gold salts, 34 percent responded well, 43 percent had untoward reactions necessitating discontinuing the therapy, and 23 percent simply did not respond at all. Yet when the serum gold levels of all three subgroups were checked, no significant differences were found.)

Gold salts are not properly used until other, more conservative modes of treatment have been tried and found wanting. Nor are they employed in a remission period. Only if there is persistent, continuing pain and inflammation, with advancing joint destruction, despite the broadly employed oral medications discussed in the next chapter, is gold indicated. Then, most rheumatologists agree, gold therapy should be instituted— with great caution.

That means beginning with very low doses, gradually increasing the dose and leveling off, eventually, at what has been determined is a safely tolerated maintenance dosage. Weekly injections are given for a sixteen- to twenty-week period, then every two weeks, and finally monthly; if all has gone well, the injections are continued indefinitely. All going well means, of course, that the therapy has proved both effective and safe for the individual patient. Improvement—retarding of the inflammatory process and diminution of pain—will generally not be evident until three or four months have gone by, since at the initial low dosages, it will take that long for a therapeutic level to be attained.

Meanwhile, from the start, both patient and doctor must watch for signs of untoward reactions. Each visit to the doctor's office must include thorough examination; frequent laboratory tests, including complete blood counts, checking of the sed rate, urinalysis, and liver-function assays, must be done. The patient, between visits, must be alert for, and instantly report to the physician, these key trouble signals: rash and/or itching, clear evidence of allergic reaction; unexplained soreness anywhere, especially in the mouth; "indigestion" or other gastrointestinal difficulties or departures from usual patterns; jaundice, or yellowing of the skin or whites of the eyes.

Surgery. As we noted earlier, there has been increasing interest in, and heartening success with, surgical procedures. This has been especially true in rheumatoid arthritis. Three kinds of procedures, in particular, have been proving useful.

One is synovectomy, removal of the synovial membrane enveloping a joint. In RA, a major cause of pain and of joint damage as well is that the synovium becomes inflamed, thickens, and releases great numbers of lysosomal enzymes (see pages 7–8) into the joint, leading eventually to destruction of cartilage and bone. Synovectomy, performed early in the course of the disease, can prevent a good deal of that, affording welcome relief from pain and discomfort; in one major study involving synovectomies performed on the finger joints of 121 successive patients, over 90 percent experienced notable relief, and four out of five reported *complete* relief. The synovium does eventually grow back, but the new membrane is of course far less inflamed—and the operation can, if necessary, be repeated.

A second sort of surgery is arthroplasty, the total joint replacement we talked about in Chapter 5 (page 74). In RA, that type of procedure has been useful not only for larger joints, i.e., hips and knees, but for finger and knuckle joints as well. In the latter, reconstructions employing silastic (inert silicone rubber) implants have achieved marked improvement in flexibility and virtual transformation of severe deformities. Most recently, silastic membrane arthroplasty has also proved a promising technique for wrist reconstruction, particularly when RA has caused destruction of the small bones of the joint.

The third, most widely applicable to the wrist, is fusion—complete immobilization of the joint. While that may seem contradictory (isn't that what we want to *prevent?*), it isn't really. When the disease process itself results in joint immobility, it typically takes a distorted form: the wrist is often twisted sharply to one side; the muscles surrounding the joint are in continual painful spasm and greatly weakened; the hand is not only unsightly but virtually useless. Even when no deformity has occurred, weakness and loss of dexterity, coupled with pain on joint movement, can make the performance of everyday tasks impossible.

The wrist-fusion procedure, called arthrodesis (from the Greek *desis*, "binding together"), can often provide an answer to these multiple problems. In the operation, the back of the wrist is opened; scar tissue, synovium, and damaged bone and cartilage are removed; and a long metal pin, extending from the base of the fingers up into the radius (one of the two bones of the forearm), is inserted with the wrist aligned with the forearm in a "neutral" position. Results, in the operations that have been performed, have been quite impressive.

An illustrative series of fusions was performed at the Robert B. Brigham Hospital in Boston (an institution devoted entirely to arthritic and rheumatic disorders), and reported to a meeting of the American Rheumatism Association in 1972. Among the patients who elected to undergo the procedure, 48 percent sought relief from the constant pain resulting from motion; 17 percent exhibited definite deformities; 35 percent, while they were not conscious of pain, had marked loss of hand strength (due, their physicians concluded, primarily to instinctive disuse of muscles in order to prevent pain). Results of the reported cases: diminution or complete loss of pain, consistent increase in hand strength (the shoulder and elbow joints easily provide needed rotation) and renewed ability to perform everyday tasks; plus, of course, a restored normal appearance in those wrists in which deformity had occurred.

Emotional Components? In some cases, physicians have observed that RA can worsen under, or flare-ups can be triggered by, emotional stress. Sometimes the stress can lead to unwise physical activity that is, in turn, the direct precipitator of the flare-up; in other instances, the cause-and-effect connection is more obscure. The possibility of such a relationship is, at any rate, often worth entertaining; a great number of RA sufferers have found that psychotherapy that reduces anxieties has helped to diminish the frequency and severity of flare-ups as well.

Juvenile Rheumatoid Arthritis (JRA)

If anything, juvenile rheumatoid arthritis is even more mystical in origin—and difficult to diagnosis—than the adult variety. It may even, in fact, be two (or more) different diseases.

JRA can apparently occur as serious illness, coming on rather suddenly with fairly high fever, a measleslike rash, and very little joint involvement. It is then often termed *Still's Disease* (sometimes a term applied to any form of JRA). Or its onset may be much like that of adult RA—rather gradual, with progressive joint pain and destruction. In the first type, patients typically lack the *rheumatoid factor* that characterizes 75 percent of adult RA patients; there is also often enlargement of the spleen and lymph nodes (findings generally denoting acute infection). This acute type may be self-limited—disappearing within weeks, months, or years, with or without specific treatment.

Current thinking postulates that the prior line between juvenile and adult RA may not have been correctly drawn. It is possible that the conditions—whether the victim is child or adult—are two different diseases, and that one may be acute and the other chronic, whatever the age of onset. A number of cases—in adults—have in fact been reported that seemed to follow a classic acute "JRA" pattern, with intense activity, lack of the rheumatoid factor, and a spontaneous "burning itself out," as the spontaneous total remission has often been described. There have been, on the other hand, many instances of "juvenile" (because the patients were children) RA that followed a typical adult pattern, eventually becoming the classic chronic kind of disabling disease.

We do not seem to be offering much of a definitive nature to the reader. Unfortunately—despite what has been written elsewhere—there is little of a definitive nature to offer. We simply cannot yet tell you whether your child who has been diagnosed as having JRA is likely to outgrow it or not, certainly if the onset has occurred before the age of six (there is statistically a one-in-three chance); if the condition has persisted into (or has first occurred in) the teens, it is highly likely to be equivalent to adult RA.

The more powerful anti-inflammatory drugs such as indomethacin and phenylbutazone have not been proved safe—and are therefore contraindicated—in children. Medication for JRA (probable or suspected) consists of the basic analgesics, cautious use of more potent prescription painkillers (if necessary), and/or equally cautious use of the corticosteroids, plus concomitant safeguarding of the child's general health via adequate rest, a balanced diet, and protection from infection. Gold therapy has also proved very effective in many children.

Three additional points should be noted.

One is that—as must be apparent—the diagnosis is frequently open to question, and parents in whose child JRA has been diagnosed may wish to seek a second opinion, since interpretation of clinical data, even when that data has been read accurately, may vary. Among some conditions that can present uncannily similar pictures, to mention just a few, are injury (which the child may not recall); localized infection within the joint; systemic infections, including rheumatic fever; a variety of neuromuscular conditions such as muscular dystrophy; certain allergic reactions; other arthritic disorders such as SLE and dermatomyositis; leukemia; and hereditary blood disorders such as hemophilia and sickle-cell anemia. There are also a number of other problems afflicting children, including Legg-Perthes Disease, a self-limited degeneration of the growing end of a long bone, which results in pain in the joint (*or* in another joint) and requires complete rest of the affected joint for a period varying from several months to two years; an expert can detect the last condition on X ray.

The second is the question of administration of rubella (German measles) vaccine to a child with JRA. There has been a high degree of suspicion, among rheumatologists, that there may be a connection between the two diseases; an unusually high level of rubella antibodies has been detected in many youngsters with long-standing JRA. And in a child with JRA, rubella vaccination can aggravate the condition, with extremely uncomfortable results for the child. Therefore, rubella vaccination for a child with active JRA should be postponed until the condition has been in remission for an extended period.

The third is that, for reasons unknown, a serious eye condition called iridocyclitis—an inflammation of both the iris and certain adjacent structures of the eyeball—occurs in approximately 15 percent of JRA victims. It is typically not visibly evident, but a simple blood test for the presence of substances called antinuclear antibodies can help to identify most of those who are likely to develop the condition. Treatment, including steroids, is necessary to prevent scarring that may lead to visual loss. Thus, parents of a child with JRA are urged to be sure the youngster receives appropriate testing at periodic intervals. (Studies suggest that iridocyclitis is highly unlikely to occur in those JRA patients who evidence the rheumatoid factor.)

Ankylosing Spondylitis (AS)

Let's get through the definitions quickly. The *-itis* is of course inflammation. *Spondylos*, from the Greek word for "vertebra." *Ankylosis*, again Greek, meaning "stiffening of a joint"—although the stiffening is not necessarily inevitable now. It's also known variably as Marie's Disease or Marie-Strümpell Disease, depending upon what physician(s) one wishes to credit for noting its existence. More and more, we are referring to it simply as rheumatoid spondylitis, probably the most accurate term.

What it is: essentially an RA-like arthritis of the spine,

tending typically to stiffen or immobilize that series of joints, that is—except for its specific location—very similar to rheumatoid arthritis. Unlike the situation with the other arthritic disorders (except for gout), there is a distinct preponderance of male patients—possibly ten to one—so that it is suspected that there is a hereditary factor, at least in predisposing to the condition (and multiple cases in families are often seen). The causative agent is completely unknown, but may be similar to that of RA.

AS principally involves the lower spine at first, but may affect nearby joints—such as the hips and shoulders—as well; other joints, such as the hands or feet, are very rarely involved. It typically begins with pain in the lower back, and the characteristic stiffness may progress upward until the spine is for all intents and purposes totally rigid, with the victim walking about quite stiffly—sometimes, with a forced "stoop" of the back.

Ankylosing spondylitis, unlike RA, seems to be a self-limited disorder; it comes to a spontaneous halt after a few years. But whatever deformity or stiffness has been perpetrated during its course remains. Thus, the aim of therapy is the prevention or minimizing of such lasting effects.

It is especially young men, between the teens and the early forties, who are attacked by AS; 80 percent of the five hundred thousand to one million victims are in fact under thirty-five. The early pain in the lower back is generally fairly mild and occasional, and may take one of several forms. Most commonly, there is muscle spasm, the type of twinge that used to be called "lumbago." In some cases, it is much like osteoarthritis in that the back is stiff and achy after prolonged periods of rest (as when arising in the morning) and improves after moving about for a while. The third kind of backache that can, less commonly, characterize early AS is a radiating pain that shoots down one leg or—confusingly—into the abdomen; this type typically occurs at night. While the discomfort is more or less continuous for about one in four patients, in most it follows a flare-up-and-remission pattern much like that of RA, with the remission periods lasting for weeks, months, or even years.

Diagnosis can be difficult, since manifestations are detectable by X ray in fewer than half those afflicted by AS even after as long as five years; in some, the period may be ten years or longer. (Once stiffening *has* occurred—usually accompanied by the postural changes we mentioned earlier, as well as compression of the chest and breathing difficulty, the diagnosis is very obvious; the damage has been done—although sometimes surgery, combined with other rehabilitative measures, can effect dramatic improvement.) Nor are laboratory tests, so helpful in RA, necessarily of use in AS; there is no special "factor," and the erythrocyte sedimentation rate that is consistently elevated in almost all RA patients is perfectly normal in one in five of those suffering from AS.

Certainly if particular changes in the spine are pinpointed on X ray, and the sed rate is elevated as well, there will be no doubt of the diagnosis. But even if AS is merely suspected, rheumatologists agree that therapy is desirable, and the sooner the better, not only in order to relieve pain but to prevent or at least minimize damage and possible deformity and to promote mobility and optimal posture.

Treatment. A number of the basic anti-inflammatory medications discussed in Chapter 7 have been found useful in AS. These include the salicylates—aspirin and family—as well as the more potent analgesics such as indomethacin, phenylbutazone, and oxyphenbutazone; the latter are employed particularly during periods of flare-up and increased inflammation. Muscle relaxants (they are among those drugs known as "minor tran-quilizers," and include Librium, Serax, and Valium) are often helpful, too, since they counter the pain of muscular spasm as well as the exacerbation of spinal inflammation that can result from muscular strain and tension. The corticosteroids are very rarely needed or used in AS, and the gold-salts therapy that has had such success in RA has not at this writing been proved effective for spondylitis.

As important in AS as drugs to fight inflammation is a program of rest and physical therapy. Any activities that strain, twist, or distort the spine must be avoided—while heat, massage, and just plain flat-on-the-back rest are quite valuable. At the same time, special exercises and postural training can help to strengthen the torso muscles and prevent future deformity (a back brace may also sometimes be used for brief periods). We shall comment further on this regimen in Chapter 8.

SEVEN

The Medicine Cabinet

In Chapters 3 through 6, we have gone into considerable detail about a number of specific drugs that have proved helpful in specific arthritic disorders—the antimalarials and immunosuppressives in SLE; colchicine, probenecid, sulfinpyrazone, and allopurinol in gout; gold salts in rheumatoid arthritis. We have also repeatedly referred the reader to this chapter. Here, we shall talk about the broadly useful antipain and anti-inflammation medications, both those available over the drugstore counter and those requiring a physician's prescription.

They fall, roughly, into five categories: aspirin and other over-the-counter pain and inflammation relievers; the more potent prescription anti-inflammatories; powerful drugs that act primarily to block pain; relaxants and sedatives; and the corticosteroids, hormones that help to bolster the body's withstanding of stress. These five classes of medications form the heart of the arthritis pharmacopoeia. Some are in a sense almost wonder workers, when properly employed. Improperly or carelessly used, some can unquestionably wreak havoc.

This may be, in our view, the most important chapter of this book. We believe the arthritis patient owes himself or herself a knowledge of the facts—facts that one's own physician may not have time to relate.

97

Know Your Medication . . .

More and more physicians are moving to the position that prescriptions should be precisely labeled—not only with dosage and frequency of administration, but with the precise name of the drug: the generic name and the trade name as well, if applicable. We agree entirely. Ask your doctor to so specify on the prescription form. Do *not* accept a pharmacist's protest that "such information cannot be put on a label." That is simply not true. By law, a pharmacist must put on the label *whatever the physician directs*. Which means, quite specifically, that if the physician writes "LABEL" on the prescription form—which means "label with name and dosage"—then the pharmacist had better spell out precisely that. By precisely, we mean, for example, "Indocin (indomethacin), 25 mg" or "Medrol (methylprednisolone), 16 mg" or "Talwin (pentazocine), 50 mg"; such designations as "anti-inflammatory," "corticosteroid," or "analgesic" are not sufficient.

Why have we made such a point of this? There are several reasons.

One is that you will be able to read intelligently, understand, and absorb the kind of information we present in this chapter.

A second is that discussions with physicians are greatly facilitated. If you have telephoned the doctor who is treating your arthritic condition to report that the medication has failed to lessen your discomfort, or that you have experienced an untoward side effect, and you are asked, "What is your medication schedule now?" it will not be very helpful if your answer is "I take those blue capsules twice a day," or "I'm on those little yellow pills."

Further, if you are consulting a different doctor for a different condition, it is vital—because of potentially hazardous interactions between certain drugs—that you be able to tell that doctor exactly what medications you are currently taking.

Finally, a clearly labeled container protects others, as well. A number of the medications we shall mention can be lethal in unusually large amounts, whether taken accidentally or deliberately—and the risk rises in inverse proportion to the size of the individual. If your toddler has just gulped down the entire contents of a bottle of medication, precious moments can be saved when you phone your physician or your local poison control center if you can immediately name the drug.

. . . And Follow These Five Rules

It is wise, again for the protection of both patient and other people, to follow these five very basic principles. They are simple, uncomplicated, and easy to adhere to; many a complication has resulted from ignoring them.

1. Follow your physician's directions as to dosage and schedule of medication, implicitly. Medication in the arthritic disorders is often a tricky, trial-and-error matter at best, as we noted earlier. If you deviate from your doctor's recommendations, then neither you nor your doctor can come to a rational conclusion concerning the effectiveness of the medicine.

This holds true whether you are taking a prescription drug, an over-the-counter product, or both. Remember that it may be serving a prophylactic purpose; don't forget to take it on schedule, whether or not you experience any pain or discomfort. Should you feel that the amount or frequency of the medication isn't sufficient, that it is not providing adequate relief, don't take it upon yourself to boost the amount; call your doctor—who may give you new instructions as to dose and frequency, or may feel that an entirely new medication is called for, and may ask to see you for a reevaluation.

2. Any untoward effects whatever, whether or not we have mentioned them (in this chapter or in comments in prior chapters), mean that you should stop the medication and contact your doctor *immediately*. Bleeding, interference with vital functions such as respiration, or neurological symptoms (visual difficulty or impairment, for instance, or loss of muscular control or coordination) are obvious alarm signals. But less terrifying developments, whatever they may be—headache, gastrointestinal oddities, any unexpected sign or sensation, no matter how seemingly minor—qualify as well.

3. Consult your doctor before taking *any other medication*. Drugs can interact, broadly speaking, in one of two ways.

One substance can potentiate—increase or "boost"—the effects of the other. In some instances, this can be a mutual effect, what is technically termed *synergistic*: i.e., the combination is more powerful than simple additive effects would lead one to expect. Sometimes this is desirable, and the synergistic effect is deliberately exploited, as in the combination of certain antibiotics in combating some infections, or of ergotamine and caffeine in treating migraine headache. Often it is not, as in the combination of some sedatives and tranquilizers with alcohol; that particular combination—of amounts of each that would have in themselves been innocuous—has killed a great many people.

Or therapeutic effects can be reduced or negated—again, in a one-way or two-way pattern; several such effects, involving special medications for gout, were noted in Chapter 4. Other examples: the therapeutic benefits of some analgesics and anti-inflammatory drugs are canceled by some barbiturate sedatives; some drugs designed to lower blood cholesterol may interfere with the absorption of aspirin; there is experimental evidence that aspirin inhibits the therapeutic effect of indomethacin.

Earlier, we referred to the necessity of telling one doctor what another has prescribed. We repeat that admonition. If you consult, let us say, an ear-nose-and-throat specialist for a sinus problem, be sure to let that physician know about current medication for an arthritic condition, whatever it may be. Conversely, when you consult a doctor about an arthritic problem, be sure to mention any *other* disorder—e.g., a heart or circulatory problem, high blood pressure, diabetes—and the medication you take for it, as well as any other physical condition, such as pregnancy, that may have a bearing on medication safety.

We've been referring chiefly to prescription drugs, but this precaution holds for over-the-counter drugs as well, a fact of which many people are unfortunately unaware. There are few labeling regulations established for such products; it is devoutly to be hoped that the situation will be remedied in future. If it is, some of the ubiquitous antacids will carry admonitions reading WARNING: THIS PRODUCT MAY INCREASE OR DECREASE THE ABSORPTION RATE OF OTHER MEDICATIONS. IF YOU ARE TAKING ANY OTHER MEDICATION, CONSULT YOUR PHYSICIAN BEFORE USING THIS PRODUCT.

In short, don't mix drugs, no matter how innocuous they may seem to be, without discussing the question with your doctor(s).

4. As we suggested a little earlier, medications of any type can be very dangerous when it comes to small children—who are historically prone to gobble down almost anything. Children under the age of five account for 82 percent of all cases of aspirin poisoning in our nation, and one out of five cases of

child poisoning in this age group is accounted for by aspirin. Prescription drugs, obviously, pose an enhanced danger.

Containers resistant to opening by under-five children were federally mandated for aspirin and potent liniments as of January 1973; substances listed as "controlled drugs," including amphetamines, barbiturates, and preparations containing large amounts of codeine, came under the same regulation. *All* oral prescription medications, with few exceptions (none of the prescription drugs discussed in this book are excepted), must be so packaged by April, 1974. If you have children under five in your home, do be sure that such drugs are packaged in child-resistant containers—and just to be on the safe side ("resistance" is based on broadly representative tests), make sure that the container does, in fact, resist *your* child's attempts to open it.

If in doubt, keep the medication under lock and key.

5. If your physician has prescribed very potent painkillers or sedatives, and you have teen-agers or young adults in your family (or if you employ such individuals as baby-sitters), it is a good idea to keep these medications locked away; extensive abuse has been reported with all the barbiturates, as well as with a number of the potent analgesics and nonbarbiturate sedatives.

Over the Counter: Aspirin and Other Analgesics

Aspirin is probably the most useful medication in existence. Chemically acetylsalicylic acid, it was first synthesized in 1899; its name comes from *a*cetyl and *spir*aeic acid, the former name for salicylic acid.

We still do not understand, after all these years, just how aspirin works. We know that it relieves pain, it lowers fever, and it reduces inflammation—all without producing dependence or affecting behavior or mental processes. There is increasing evidence that at least part of its action takes place in the realm of the prostaglandins (more about this recently identified group of substances in Chapter 11). It is, at any rate, *the* basic "drug of choice" for all types of arthritis with the single exception of gout. (And aspirin should not, in fact, be taken by someone with gout who is on probenecid or sulfinpyrazone therapy, since it inhibits the action of those uricosurics.)

What, then, of that mysterious unnamed substance that "doctors recommend most" you have seen advertised? Actually, what the makers of Anacin are talking about *is* aspirin, and doctors *do* recommend it most. They do not recommend Anacin, however, since they do not see the need for you to pay for that advertising, or for the other ingredient in the product, which happens to be caffeine. Caffeine is the mild stimulant present in coffee, tea, and cola; if you feel you need some pepping up along with your pain relief, it is a lot cheaper to take some aspirin and drink a cup of coffee.

While caffeine is helpful, as we noted earlier, in the treatment of migraine headache, it is totally irrelevant as an ingredient in products intended for other types of pain. It may even, in fact, be definitely harmful. As Drs. William H. Barr and Richard P. Penna, writing in the American Pharmaceutical Association's *Handbook of Non-Prescription Drugs* (1971), have pointed out: "Caffeine has a variety of pharmacological effects unrelated to analgesia. . . . Preparations containing caffeine may be inadvisable for certain persons with nervous disorders or cardiovascular conditions. The use of compounds containing caffeine also is not advisable for rheumatoid or other conditions requiring large doses (10 to 30 tablets daily) where caffeine toxicities actually could be encountered. The increased hydrochloric acid production caused by caffeine may also aggravate the gastrointestinal damage produced by aspirin in persons taking large or frequent doses."

Nor are other combination products of particular value, despite their claims of "faster" relief, "extra strength," and the like. If you check the very small type on packages of such products—as, Bufferin, Empirin Compound, Excedrin, Vanquish, etc.—you will find that they variously contain such ingredients, in addition to aspirin, as salicylamide, acetaminophen, phenacetin, and/or such mouthfuls as aluminum hydroxide and magnesium carbonate. The first three are other analgesics. Salicylamide has been proved inferior to aspirin, and its efficacy is not enhanced in combination. Acetaminophen is a useful analgesic, but has no anti-inflammatory properties, hence may be helpful in conditions not involving inflammation, meaning occasionally in osteoarthritis; it is available all by itself under a number of trade names (Tempra, Tylenol, Valadol, et al.). Phenacetin, which does not combat inflammation either, is an otherwise effective but risky analgesic suspected of perpetrating kidney damage in some instances (products including it are required by law to carry a warning) and anemia in others; some believe that combining it with aspirin may potentiate its toxic effects. You may find, too, that these products contain *less* than the standard amount of aspirin (300 to 325 milligrams per tablet)—which is what your doctor wants you to have unless otherwise specified.

Those other components with the lengthy names are found on the products that claim to be "faster acting" and promise "no stomach upset." It's true that aspirin can sometimes cause the latter difficulty. But it's not true that these extra ingredients, which are various antacids, deliver either benefit. The

Food and Drug Administration has flatly termed Bufferin's advertised claims "misleading"; many medical experts have used far harsher words. (Comparative studies, in fact, have shown that both aspirin in effervescent solution—Alka-Seltzer—and ordinary aspirin taken with hot water have faster absorption rates than buffered aspirin. Alka-Seltzer should not, however, be used for continued or prolonged analgesic purposes, since its antacid content could well precipitate a type of chemical imbalance called alkalosis.)

There remain some single-ingredient products we haven't commented on. Other salicylates, such as calcium carbaspirin (Calurin), choline salicylate (Arthropan), and sodium salicylate, like salicylamide, simply are not as effective as aspirin. There are also other forms of aspirin itself. Specially coated tablets (e.g., Ecotrin) may be helpful when there is demonstrated gastrointestinal sensitivity, but their absorption rate is both slow and unpredictable. Some aspirins now come in higher dosages promoted as of "arthritic strength"; they should be used only on a physician's recommendation. Measurin, Cama, and other time-release aspirins can be of great aid as overnight medication in conditions that involve either severe morning stiffness or the possibility of pain that can occur and awaken you during the night. But the use of *any* form other than regular, standard-dosage aspirin tablets should be first discussed with your physician.

Now, how about those drawbacks? Aspirin does have some. While it's an extremely valuable medication, it's not perfect; no drug is. One difficulty can be the gastrointestinal sensitivity we mentioned, which some people do have. It stems both from mechanical irritation and stimulated acid production, and can frequently be minimized by taking the aspirin either immediately after a meal or with a glass of milk. Another is the fact that some people are allergic to aspirin, and if that sort of reaction (often first manifested by a rash) has occurred, further taking of it isn't advisable. Nor is aspirin—especially in the heavy and continuing regimen often required in arthritic disorders—considered advisable in those suffering from bleeding disorders, heart conditions requiring anticoagulants, or peptic ulcer.

Lastly, even if none of the foregoing obtain, continuing aspirin administration over a period of time can give rise to a variety of inimical effects, symptomized notably by ringing in the ears, headache, profuse sweating, nervousness, gastrointestinal upset, or black or near-black stools (which signify bleeding in the gastrointestinal tract resulting from serious irritation); should such signs appear, the physician will generally direct that the dosage be reduced, or that the patient stop taking the drug, at least temporarily.

It is when one of the foregoing situations obtains, as well as when aspirin does not seem to be performing well for an individual patient, that the physician will turn to the prescription pharmacopoeia—the four groups of drugs that follow.

The Potent Anti-Inflammatories

These are the drugs to which the physician may turn in periods of acute inflammation, when pain is severe and the potential for joint damage great. They have been found helpful in gout, osteoarthritis, rheumatoid arthritis, and spondylitis. They are extremely powerful drugs, both for good and for ill. While they can offer rapid relief of pain, they also present many risks similar to those of aspirin—except that they can occur more quickly and can be far more serious—plus a number of other potential perils.

Thus, they are properly used only for very brief periods, which we shall specify. Thus, too, it is extremely important for someone taking any of these medications to be alert for signs of untoward reactions. And because the possibility of gastrointestinal irritation and ulcer creation is markedly higher than with aspirin (all three of these drugs are flatly contraindicated in those with a history of gastrointestinal inflammation of any sort), they should *always* be taken following a meal or with a glass of milk.

All three drugs are also contraindicated (not proved safe, thus deemed inadvisable) in pregnancy, in nursing mothers, and in children under the age of fourteen.

The first of the three is indomethacin (Indocin), which was initially introduced for the treatment of flare-up in rheumatoid arthritis. It is actually about as effective as aspirin for that condition—and is not an alternative in case of allergy to aspirin, since there is a cross-sensitivity (i.e., someone allergic to one is likely to react similarly to the other), even though indomethacin is not a salicylate. It is, however, extremely effective in acute phases of gout, in osteoarthritis of the knee or hip exacerbated by inflammation, and in spondylitis.

The time period for administration of indomethacin may vary a good deal with the individual patient's reactions. Typically, the physician will begin with an extremely low dosage and will gradually increase it until relief is achieved or side effects are manifested, whichever happens first; generally a few weeks is the outside limit. In the meantime, it's quite important to watch for some of those problems.

One area, as we've already mentioned, is gastrointestinal irritation; indications of that might be abdominal pain, or very dark stools, suggesting bleeding somewhere in the tract. The reverse, unusually light stools, should also serve as an alarm signal, indicating possible liver problems. Hair loss may occur; it's reversible, and certainly not lethal—but it is a sign of adverse reaction. There may also be neurological reactions. Severe or persistent headache should be a cause for concern, as should hearing difficulty or vision problems (in particular, blurred vision, extended dark-adaptation time, or color-vision abnormalities); the vision defects often persist for a while, even months, after the drug is stopped, but they do disappear eventually. Any of these symptoms, as well as any other unexplained sensation (undue fatigue, for example) should be reported to the doctor without delay.

The other two drugs in this category are closely related ones called butazones: phenylbutazone (Butazolidin, Azolid) and oxyphenbutazone (Tandearil, Oxalid). They can be quite helpful for flare-ups in gout, rheumatoid arthritis, and spondylitis. They are, however, even more potent than indomethacin; they are not the preferred drugs for these conditions, and the course of therapy should not last longer than a few days, a week at most. In addition to what we've said earlier, contraindications include previously established allergy; liver, heart, or kidney dysfunction; a tendency to water retention; circulatory disorders, including high blood pressure; the very elderly; peptic ulcer; and anyone taking any other potent medication, including—but not only—an anticoagulant.

The butazones are capable of triggering trouble in a number of ways. Someone taking them should be especially alert for, and report promptly to the doctor: fever; sore throat or mouth sores; any urinary or gastrointestinal departures or abnormalities, including very light or very dark stools; nausea; a rash or any other skin reaction; reddish or purplish bruiselike spots appearing in the absence of injury (suggesting spontaneous hemorrhage into the skin, medically called *purpura*); sudden weight

gain; swelling anywhere in the body. Additionally, the butazones can potentiate—i.e., boost the effects of—both insulin
and the oral drugs taken for diabetes; if you are a diabetic, it is
vital to be especially alert for incipient insulin reaction when
you are on butazone therapy.

The Powerful Analgesics

Opiates—codeine, meperidine (Demerol), and the like—are
very rarely, if ever, prescribed for the arthritic disorders. Three
other drugs that are not officially classed as dangerous (they
are termed, technically, "noncontrolled narcotics") sometimes
are. They are propoxyphene (Darvon), pentazocine (Talwin),
and ethoheptazine (Zactane).

The main thing of which the patient should be aware is the
fact that these drugs are, actually, potentially addictive. Which
means that the physician's instructions must be adhered to very
carefully. None can be considered safe for pregnant women,
nursing mothers, or children.

We hasten to add that continuing low dosages have usually
not proved addictive in ordinary use as prescribed. That "as
prescribed" is important. If a particular dosage at particular intervals is directed, follow it. Needless to say, these drugs must
be kept away from anyone who might be tempted to misuse or
abuse them.

Our basic advice is to use these drugs minimally—if possible,
even to a lesser degree than your prescription might permit.
Unlike aspirin, indomethacin, and the butazones, they are not
designed to diminish inflammation or other troublemaking conditions, but simply to relieve pain. Thus, it is not important
to take them like clockwork, on a particular schedule; use them,

if your doctor has prescribed them, when you know they are needed.

There are, as with most drugs, side effects (unrelated to dependence) that should mean an immediate report to the physician; they may affect, especially, the central nervous system, circulation, and the gastrointestinal tract. Alarm signals that mean a call to the doctor is in order: dizziness; nausea; headache; constipation; weakness; insomnia; visual difficulties of any kind; chills or sweating; any rash or itching, suggesting allergy.

It should be noted that an intensive Mayo Clinic study, reported in 1972, concluded that propoxyphene and ethoheptazine are inferior to ordinary aspirin in pain-relief potential. They may, however, be useful in situations in which aspirin is contraindicated for some reason.

None of these drugs should be combined with alcohol.

Relaxants and Sedatives

These drugs are used more widely in psychosomatic conditions than in arthritic disorders; they may, however, be employed if the physician judges that it is advisable, particularly those "tranquilizers" or sedatives that incorporate muscle-relaxant properties. We earlier mentioned that such properties may be especially useful in spondylitis, which can be badly aggravated by muscle spasm; such spasm can of course play a part in osteoarthritis and in rheumatoid arthritis as well.

Included among the drugs generally termed sedatives are those commonly called "tranquilizers," as well as the barbiturates and other sleep promoters. Those incorporating the muscle-relaxant properties that can be useful in arthritic conditions include, prominently, carisoprodol (Soma)—which is basically an analgesic—and several of the so-called "minor tranquilizers," particularly chlordiazepoxide (Librium), oxáze-pam (Serax), and diazepam (Valium); the last is especially employed for its muscle-relaxant properties.

Be advised, because it's vital, that the "tranquilizing" medications do have habit-forming potential. Not, admittedly, to the extent that propoxyphene, pentazocine, and ethoheptazine do—but the potential is there nonetheless. This means that it is vital that the prescribed regimen be adhered to, and not exceeded as to either dosage or frequency.

Potential adverse reactions to these medications are so variable that it would take another half book, at least, to list them. Let us simply say that *any* unexpected symptom *whatever* should be instantly reported to the doctor. And another precaution: never combine tranquilizers or sedatives with alcohol, or with any other psychoactive or potentially habit-forming drug (including the aforementioned powerful analgesics, sleeping pills whether barbiturates or not, antidepressants, other tranquilizers, "diet pills," or medication for any neurological disorder such as epilepsy).

The Corticosteroids

They are sometimes referred to simply as "corticoids." Their full name, which nobody uses, is "adrenocorticosteroids." They are natural hormones, or synthetic versions thereof; they are very powerful, very effective, and potentially very dangerous. They are used—if the physician judges them to be necessary—in most of the arthritic diseases, with some exceptions: they are not considered advisable in gout; they are only very rarely used in scleroderma or in spondylitis; and they are not used in osteoarthritis, with the sole exception that they may, as we mentioned in Chapter 5, occasionally be injected directly into a painful joint.

To backtrack for a moment. Two of the vital endocrine glands in the body are the pair called the adrenal glands. The cortex, or outer part, of these glands secretes, in humans, a substance called cortisol. (Some other mammals secrete, in their adrenal glands, a similar hormone called cortisone. Cortisone, when administered to a human being, is converted to cortisol—so for all intents and purposes, we are talking about the same thing.) So far, we've explained "adreno" and "cortico." The "steroid"—or sterol-like—part stems from something of interest chiefly to chemists: that these substances have a chemical structure similar to that of cholesterol.

There are now a number of versions of these chemicals that have been synthesized, and we are not going to list them all or even the majority of them. Generic terms include, in addition to those we've mentioned, prednisone, prenisolone, methylprednisolone, triamcinolone, and more. Trade names include Aristocort, Cortone, Decadron, Deltasone, Deronil, Gammacorten, Kenacort, Medrol, Meticorten, Paracort, Sterane, and many, many more. A great many physicians feel that the trade-named preparations are in no way superior to the generic designations, although they can cost the patient from thirty to forty times as much (prednisone, at this writing, runs about two cents per tablet; certain of the brand-named products can actually cost as much as eighty cents).

What cortisol does, in the ordinary course of events, is pitch in and help the body to withstand assorted types of physical stress, which may be caused by a variety of things including hostile climatic conditions, wounds, toxic substances, or attacks by infectious organisms. One reason for giving substitutes is failure—or mandated removal—of the adrenal glands. Administered in *addition* to the body's normal supplies, the effect of the corticosteroids is to suppress or control symptoms (these drugs, it should be emphasized, do *not* directly combat the basic cause of the problem). They are used not only in those conditions with which we are dealing, but also in certain instances of respiratory distress, extreme allergic reactions, some toxic animal bites for which there is no antidote, etc.

In the arthritic disorders, the effects of the corticosteroids are often dramatic. Pain, and inflammation as well, may be rapidly suppressed. The patient may well "feel good again" in short order. Long-term regimens have also proved effective. They are frequently used on a prophylactic "maintenance" basis, for fairly extended periods, when RA patients, for example, have proved hypersensitive to aspirin and similar drugs. They have also been unusually successful in children with dermatomyositis, who have often totally recovered—the disease having "run its course"—within a two-year period, "tided over" by corticosteroids.

Unfortunately, the adverse effects of these drugs can be as dramatic as the beneficial ones, since they do interfere with bodily responses to a variety of stimuli. We could not possibly list them all; part of the problem is that those taking them respond highly individually. But the patient who is taking them should know that among documented effects are: growth retardation in children (more likely with the synthetics than with the natural substances); disruption of menstrual schedules; slowed hair growth; slowed healing of minor injuries; masking of symptoms of acute infections; aggravation of high blood pressure, emotional problems, or peptic ulcer; facial swelling ("moonface"); muscular weakness; gastrointestinal upsets; easy bruisability.

Physicians are all very much aware of these problems. The

corticosteroids are never first-choice medications; they are reserved for patients and situations in whom or which there have been severe problems and lack of response to other therapy. The dosages are kept as low as possible—i.e., the physician will seek to establish the minimum effective dosage for the individual patient—since the side effects are always *cumulative*; the lower the dosage, the less likely that side effects will occur. Frequently the drug will be prescribed on an every-other-day basis. Invariably, the patient will be taken off corticosteroid therapy as soon as possible. The physician will make every effort to avoid prescribing these drugs at all if the patient is pregnant, since they have apparently been related in some cases to the birth of babies low in weight or suffering from initial respiratory difficulties.

As with the other drugs we've been discussing, it is up to the patient to report promptly to the doctor any evidence of any untoward reaction whatever. The patient should also keep some other precautions in mind:

1. A diabetic should be aware that these drugs can lower the body's ability to cope with carbohydrates; a change in insulin or other hypoglycemic drug dosage may be in order, and the question should be discussed with the doctor.

2. Fungal infections should be swiftly revealed to the doctor prescribing corticosteroids, if he or she is not aware of them (if, say, they are being treated by another physician); they are a contraindication for corticosteroids.

3. Vaccinations are contraindicated while on corticosteroid therapy; there are hazards of overwhelming infection, as well as neurological complications.

4. Don't take aspirin—or any similar medication—while on a corticosteroid regimen unless the drug and dosage have been fully discussed with your doctor.

5. Finally, this extremely important facet of the complexity of corticosteroid therapy: these drugs suppress the body's own natural production of adrenal hormones. When the drug is withdrawn, there is a "catch-up" period before normal function is resumed. Anyone taking such medication should (a) carry a warning card in case of accident, so that emergency medical personnel will be aware of the situation; (b) discuss the situation beforehand if surgery is contemplated for some other condition—since a lethal situation could otherwise occur on the operating table, if the surgeon is not fully informed and hormonal replacement provided. After eight weeks or more of steroid therapy, any surgery within a one-year period means that the patient should have replacement therapy.

Some readers may recall from biology courses that the pituitary gland—another endocrine gland, located within the skull —produces, among other substances, one called ACTH. The letters stand for *a*drenocorticotrophic *h*ormone, and the natural function of ACTH is the stimulation of the adrenal cortex to produce its own essential hormones. But this particular situation is different. Unfortunately, injected ACTH will not spur the adrenals to resume their activity any faster; the "catch-up" period simply cannot be cut short.

EIGHT

R & R: Rationale and Regimen

In 1966, a major conference took place under the auspices of the Division of Chronic Diseases of the U. S. Public Health Service: a series of intensive discussions titled "The Surgeon General's Workshop on Prevention of Disability from Arthritis." It brought together a number of distinguished medical and public-health professionals concerned with the problems of continuing care of victims of the various arthritic disorders—care that would prevent the loss of mobility and productivity that can sometimes ensue.

Among the major conclusions of that conference, as stated in its final report, was that "The patient's own home should be the most important facility of all in the ultimate care of the arthritic. [The home should be] an effective place for the continuation of constructive programs." The report added, noting that optimal care demands a variety of skills brought together in a "team" effort, "The patient's family physician, the patient himself, and his family are essential members of this team."

The Rs of our chapter title stand popularly for rest (or relaxation) and rehabilitation. They might also signify reassessment, reevaluation, and resolution. All play a part in the extramedical approaches to arthritis therapy. The aim, as the Surgeon General's Workshop specified, is prevention of disability—and it *is*, in the vast majority of cases, preventable.

That is something of which you should be firmly aware, if you suffer from any of the chronic arthritic conditions we have been discussing. Your doctor, your family, and you yourself can indeed do a great deal—in many everyday ways—to assure your continued functioning and to avoid the prospect of disability. In this chapter, we shall suggest some of the steps you can take. They are just that: suggestions. As we have emphasized, every individual who has arthritis is in a very definite sense unique. We hope that our thoughts will lead to still others of your own that may be especially helpful for you.

The medications and surgical techniques we've talked about in the foregoing chapters are aimed, by and large, at accomplishing two things: diminution of pain and, when necessary, correction of disability or deformity. Approaches we shall discuss in this chapter constitute not a replacement for medication, but adjunctive therapy. *Their* aims: to afford additional pain relief; to prevent aggravation of the inflammatory process that can result both in additional discomfort and in joint damage; and to avoid the possibility of deformity and/or disability. (What we shall have to say here applies to *most* types of arthritis. *Gout* is essentially a chemical problem; its inflammatory episodes are, with proper medication, short-lived.)

Before we comment on some specific areas, let's state some general assumptions. In the immediate sense, the aim of these physical steps is relief of pain and discomfort. But it is important for the arthritis sufferer to be concerned about the future, too, in two ways.

One involves the afflicted joint or joints. Anything that increases or triggers inflammation, or places additional strain on the joint, will tend to be destructive, encouraging deformity and disability. Conversely, anything that diminishes strain—that "coddles" the joint, if you will—will be helpful.

The other involves proximal structures—muscles, tendons, and so on. They should remain as strong and flexible as possible, in order to provide good support. That means strain on those structures should be avoided and, at the same time, it means strengthening routines may be in order.

We must add that all of the following should, of course, be thoroughly discussed with your own doctor.

Rest, Bed and Otherwise

There is no question that rest of an acutely inflamed joint —rest that is as close to complete as possible—is beneficial. Conversely, motion of such a joint not only increases pain, but does actual damage to the joint, as well. The first result has long been evident to arthritics. Objective evidence of the second has been lacking until recently.

But the results of a study, reported in the *Journal* of the American Medical Association in 1972, substantiated the long-standing suspicion that movement of an inflamed joint could indeed cause demonstrable damage. In that study, researchers at the University of Pennsylvania Medical School produced an "instant arthritis" in a group of dogs by injecting urate crystals into their knee joints. Each dog's right knee was then totally immobilized for a period of several hours. During that same period, the dogs' left knees were deliberately exercised for specific amounts of time—variously, five seconds, thirty seconds, five minutes, or seven and a half minutes—during each quarter hour; the rest of the time, they were kept rested in the same position as the right knees.

Results: any amount of exercise lasting for more than five

seconds per quarter hour caused what the report termed "dramatic" changes, as compared with the rested joints. Examination of the exercised joints revealed changes in the synovial membrane, dilation of blood vessels, increase in the volume of synovial fluid, and a rise in the number of leukocytes, as well as detectable cell changes—all in direct proportion to the amount of exercise. In short, there were both increased inflammatory activity and actual joint damage.

During flare-up periods, then, the affected joint(s) should be kept as rested as possible. Depending upon the part of the body involved, that may mean actual bed rest, say, if the spine or a hip is involved. Or a back brace may be recommended. For a wrist, knee, or other joint, temporary splinting may be the answer; this is an especially valuable technique in preventing deformities of the hands and fingers.

Even during remission periods, though, excessive fatigue should be avoided, since that in itself can predispose to a flare-up. Certainly that means, at the very least, adequate sleep every night—in a bed that provides both comfort and, if the spine is involved, firm support. (If you have spondylitis, you should always sleep on your back, without a pillow, in order to keep everything correctly aligned.) It should also mean the scheduling of one or two rest periods during the day, thirty- or sixty-minute periods of total relaxation, with no activity and no interruptions.

Exercise: The Good and the Bad

Basically, what you must remember if you have arthritis is not only that undue strain or stress may trigger active inflammation in an afflicted joint, but that such a joint has become more fragile, more delicate—and more subject to injury in general. Thus, any activity whatever that may place an undue burden on that joint should be carefully avoided.

If the back is involved, for example, among movements and actions to be shunned are those that involve a great deal of bending, twisting, jarring, lifting of heavy objects, or standing for prolonged periods of time—which would include sports such as golf, tennis, or horseback riding. Skiing is similarly out of the question if back, hips, knees, or ankles are affected. The single sport, in fact, that is perfectly safe and indeed recommended for someone with any kind of arthritis is swimming, preferably in a heated pool; it may, in fact, be extremely beneficial. Any other sort of activity—including hiking, cycling, or simple calisthenics—should be discussed in detail with the doctor.

The other side of the coin is that specific kinds of exercise can in fact be an extremely helpful facet of treatment. While too much exercise, or the wrong sort of exercise, can damage an arthritic joint, too *little* of the *right* sort of exercise can lead both to increased stiffness and to muscle atrophy—depriving the weakened joint of essential supporting structures and leading to impaired day-to-day functioning.

Perhaps you have seen exercises published in books on arthritis or on physical fitness generally. We have not included such routines here for a very good reason: each case is unique, and what may benefit one individual with an arthritic condition may well do irreparable damage to another suffering from the same condition. Thus, exercises self-"prescribed" from a book can well do far more harm than good. Let your physician —or a physiotherapist to whom you may be referred by your doctor—spell out the proper exercise program. We might note that this is an area where the rest of the family can help the patient immeasurably. It is best if the doctor or therapist meets not only with the patient, but with husband or wife (and in the case of a child, both parents and perhaps an older sibling as well), so that they can fully understand and actively assist in the exercise regimen.

There is also a fairly new discipline called *movement therapy*, which seeks to improve body image and function via a psychologically oriented, though basically physical, approach; it is proving increasingly promising in a variety of conditions, not limited to the arthritic disorders, that involve essentially physical problems, emotional difficulties with physical manifestations, or combinations thereof. Movement therapy is still in an experimental stage, but is attracting steadily growing support. Few individuals are as yet trained in this new modality, but if you are an arthritic patient who lives in or near a metropolitan area (where classes are at present most readily available), you might discuss the subject with your physician.

It must be added that in any involvement of the spine or hips, particularly in spondylitis, *postural* training and routines to strengthen torso muscles are essential.

Temperature and Climate

Local heat, most arthritics find, can do a great deal to relieve discomfort and stiffness. It can be applied in several ways.

One is a simple hot bath or shower—especially effective if, like many, you are afflicted with early-morning stiffness. That soothing warmth, applied on arising, can make a world of difference. Many arthritis sufferers whose *hands*, in particular, evidence such discomfort have found that wearing latex gloves during the night can help to diminish morning stiffness to a significant degree.

There are several techniques that can be used to apply heat

specifically to one or two stiff, aching joints. Inexpensive heat lamps, in the form of bulbs that can be screwed in anywhere, are widely available; they're most convenient when used with a clamp-on socket that can be attached to any piece of furniture in order to focus the heat just where it's wanted. Such a lamp should be used for about twenty minutes at a time. An electric heating pad is good for a large area such as back or hip; again, a twenty-minute period is best. A towel wrung out of hot water can also be used; cover it with plastic wrap to keep the heat in as long as possible. (When heat is being applied to a knee, ankle, or foot, do so while lying down—or sitting in a chair with the leg propped up.)

For stiff hands, try simply placing them in a basin of warm water—flexing the fingers slowly as the heat penetrates and the water cools. Or try a paraffin bath. Melt four or five pounds of paraffin in the top of a double boiler and dip the hand in several times until it's fairly thickly coated; then wrap plastic wrap around it, and a towel around that. As the wax cools and hardens, over a twenty- to thirty-minute period, the heat goes into the hand; the wax is then simply peeled off, and is reusable indefinitely. (This technique can, of course, also be used for a foot.)

Any of these techniques can be used up to two or three times a day.

How about massage? Generally it's not recommended in arthritic conditions, since forcible manipulation of an afflicted joint is anything but helpful. If the physician determines that *muscular* tension is complicating matters, however, massage treatment *may* be suggested; it should be done expertly, and only by someone the physician recommends.

Might the ministrations at one of the many spas in the United States and Europe be helpful? Yes, frequently. The

"mineral waters"—whether applied internally or externally—
will not have any effect whatever on the course of the disease;
they are in no sense curative. But warm bathing, relaxation,
and a vacation away from daily chores often constitute very
good therapy. And many spas offer the services of skilled physical therapists, as well.

Which brings us to the question of climate. If local heat generally helps, logic would dictate that atmospheric heat would
be beneficial as well—that life on the equator, perhaps, would
be blissfully arthritis-free. Unfortunately, it doesn't work that
way. Statistically, in fact, as we noted in an earlier chapter,
the incidence of rheumatoid arthritis among Eskimos is lower
than that found in inhabitants of warmer climes.

A number of studies have been done on this subject. In general, it has been found that arthritis patients tend to be affected less by the weather itself than by a sudden, radical
change in the weather—a precipitous temperature drop, for example, from 80° F. (26.6° C.) to 60° F. (15.5° C.). But temperature may actually be the least critical factor. One extensive
study carried out at the University of Wisconsin investigated
the effects of various weather components on a group of
rheumatoid arthritis patients. The consistent finding: the subjects felt *worst* not necessarily when the temperature was drop-
ping, but when the humidity was rising and/or the barometric
pressure was decreasing. Those are generally the prevailing conditions when foul weather is on the way—so those who claim
that they can "feel a storm coming" may very well be absolutely right.

It should be noted that the latter findings may not negate
the prior impressions. A descending temperature, all other
things being equal, does in fact effect a rise in the relative
humidity (what humidity is relative *to* is temperature; as the

air temperature drops, the less moisture it can hold, the more closely it approaches the "dew point," and the higher the relative humidity). But the point is that, apparently, what precipitates discomfort is the humidity rather than the temperature itself. It may be (it's simply a guess; no substantiating studies have been done) that *part* of what precipitates early-morning stiffness is the nighttime temperature drop that effects a rise in the relative humidity—the reason that dew is found on the grass in the morning.

Housework Hints

Some years ago, we might have phrased that "hints for homemakers." Meaning—that term was a euphemism—housewives. We are now well aware that those doing chores around the house may be neither wives nor women. Hence, the following tips are addressed to anyone, of either sex, who is faced with the day-to-day chores of cooking, cleaning up, and other necessary drudgery. And, of course, to areas such as home repairs and crafts.

This list is by no means complete; we hope it will stimulate your own thinking. It is based on the valid medical premises that it can only benefit the arthritic patient to avoid undue strain and sheer nuisance activity that has no therapeutic benefit, and that prior joint damage may in fact restrict or limit function. The approaches herein should be adapted to the individual's own specific needs.

–Vary your position as frequently as possible. Don't stand— or sit in one position, either—for long periods of time. If you have several tasks to accomplish, try to alternate those that require different body positions.

–If leg or hip or spinal joints are affected, plan work to cut walking up and down stairs to a minimum.

–Keep knives, saws, planes, and other cutting tools sharp; dull ones require a great deal more physical effort.

–Consider rearrangement of such areas as kitchen and workshop to make tools, cleaning supplies, and the like more accessible with less effort.

–Invest, to the limit of your financial capability, in convenience devices that can minimize physical effort on your part: an electric can opener, a mixer, a blender (which can grate, chop, and purée too), a dishwasher, a washing machine and dryer, powered craft tools.

–If you hand-wash dishes, soak them before washing. And let them air-dry rather than drying them by hand.

–Have all members of the family cooperate in cleaning chores and routine minor repairs, rather than having one responsible for all. The individual contribution takes next to no time, while one person's cleaning up after two or three or more others can be exhausting. Examples: have each clean the bathtub after using it (keep a tub brush and scouring powder handy); have anyone who notices a dirty toilet clean it (again, keep appropriate materials handy); have each individual leaving the dinner table remove his or her own plate and silverware plus one serving dish; assign overall responsibilities (taking out garbage, replacing light bulbs, regulating heat, putting family wash through the machine, etc.) to specific people. If there are a number of youngsters in the family, rotate responsibilities.

–Choose and make gadgets to render kitchen chores easier, in addition to those we've already mentioned. Examples: make vegetable-chopping a one-handed job by hammering two long rustproof nails upward through the chopping board to hold the potato, onion, or whatever; get one of the inexpensive stands that holds a cookbook open and upright, all by itself; make a wooden-rack platform to put in the kitchen sink if its present level makes for painful bending over; for peeling vegetables, use the less-strain "floating blade" type of peeler; construct a larger wooden handle that fits over your faucet, if grasping the present small one is painful or difficult.

–Take advantage of your present devices and use your imagination. If you need to tilt a bowl for mixing, and holding it in that position proves to be a strain, try this: stretch a damp dish towel over a saucepan, then place the mixing bowl (preferably a lightweight aluminum or stainless steel type) on the towel at an angle, and you'll find the traction will hold it in place. Use your kitchen stepstool for more than a stepladder: sit down to do jobs that can be done sitting down—including dishwashing. Let your roll-around vacuum cleaner give you other sitting-down opportunities; a lot can be reached with that long hose.

–Forget unnecessary tasks. Or revise your concepts of "necessary"; baby clothes don't need ironing, for example. (That task can be cut to a minimum for *all* members of the family if shoppers always look for labels that use such delightful terms as "drip dry" and "permanent press." Some of the modern synthetics are truly godsends.) Look around the house and (grit your teeth) get rid of things that are essentially useless, of little value, and mainly perpetrators of extra labor—such as elaborate dust catchers you never really cared for anyway.

–Look in all your purchases for ease of maintenance and cleaning. That means both materials and design. Sterling silver takes a lot more effort in cleaning than stainless steel. Plastic-covered upholstery is easily cleaned with soap and water or a special liquid cleaner. Lamps, vases, and other household items with intricate designs are likely to prove difficult to clean and/

or polish. Similarly, choose wall coverings that are more easily cleanable—semigloss rather than flat paint, textured plastics rather than ordinary wallpaper.

–Choose the easiest way to do anything. With the proliferation of cookbooks, there are literally thousands of tasty but easy dishes that can be substituted for a good many of the traditional but exhausting ones.

–Apply similar concepts to your own chores and household tasks, whatever they may be. Look at what you are accustomed to doing; then, ask yourself if there might not be an easier way to accomplish it—or if it might not be eliminated altogether.

NINE

Food, Drink, and
Whether to Worry About Them

The answer is no. There is no reason for anyone with arthritis to be any more concerned than anyone else with what he or she eats. There is no reason to seek out special foods or types of foods. There is no reason to shun entire categories of foods. There is no reason to take dietary supplements of any kind— vitamins, minerals, or any combination thereof—unless a physician has so directed, based upon some clear deficiency; there is, in fact, every reason not to do so, since large, unneeded dosages of certain vitamins and minerals can be not only useless, but actually toxic.

In *no* type of arthritic disorder is a special dietary regimen or menu plan required. (Even in gout, where there is a metabolic factor, no special diet is really needed; it's just a matter of avoiding a handful of certain known troublemakers, just as you would avoid strawberries, or chocolates, or peanuts, if you had a demonstrated allergy to them.) In *every* type of arthritic disorder, what is best—just as in any *non*arthritic situation—is a well-balanced, nutritious diet. You can follow all the advice in this chapter without medical consultation, whether you have an arthritic problem or not—again, unless your own doctor has specifically advised you to the contrary.

The one thing with which the arthritic patient might properly be concerned is overweight—especially in osteoarthritis, but broadly speaking in any disorder that precludes inordinate strain on the joints of the hips, knees, back, or ankles. Extra weight can be such a strain, hence additional stress upon already stressed joints. To that end, some diet modifications may be in order. But the comments we made earlier stand. Those modifications should entail neither particular additions nor particular subtractions without the benefit of medical guidance.

Some comment about the general subject of weight control is in order—in fact, is perhaps sorely needed. Hardly a month passes without some book or popular magazine's announcing, usually in bold red type, "The NEW (fill in adjective) DIET!" Such a "diet" typically places emphasis on a single food (ice cream, pickles, "natural" foods), presumably authoritatively singled out food components (high protein, low carbohydrate, high alcohol, low fat, etc.), or the weak will of the prospective readers ("Eat all you want!").

Do these "diets" work? Yes, sometimes—in the sense that weight may in fact be lost just because less is eaten. Then, you might wonder, are they not in fact good diets—at least for some people? No, they are not. If you have been gaining weight or maintaining your weight at some level above what is normal and desirable, a radical diet departure in any direction (other than simple overstuffing) is likely to effect some speedy but temporary loss. Repeat: *temporary*. A truly unusual person may switch from an ordinary diet to one consisting of pickles and wheat bran and nevertheless fail to lose weight. Most people would not; they would fairly quickly drop a number of pounds, which would as quickly return once a normal diet was resumed.

Does that mean you—or anyone—should remain on the

pickles and wheat bran, or ice cream and sesame seed, or whatever, diet? No, it does not. The warnings you have heard reiterated by reputable nutritionists are true. You *do* need a certain balance in your diet in order to keep all your body's systems functioning at an optimal level. That means—again, unless you have been so counseled by a physician—you should not take it upon yourself to exclude any group(s) of foods. If you do, you are likely to *create* serious deficiencies, along with a great many more problems than you had bargained for.

In short, all the things you have heard about the necessity of maintaining a balanced diet, incorporating all the various food groups, are absolutely true.

You can pare pounds and still maintain that balance—despite what you may have read elsewhere. Weight loss is a lot simpler than most people think it is (and many writers would *have* you think it is).

Elements and Alternates

For continued bodily functioning, you need a number of food elements. They include minerals and vitamins as well as certain other basic constituents. What is helpful is that including them does not necessarily preclude cutting calories—which are, as you may know, the weight-creating factors in food. You can, in fact, obtain those needed elements and lose weight at the same time. It depends mainly upon judicious food choices *within* the context of each source group.

Let's take protein. You've no doubt heard of it; it's a basic element in animal (including human) metabolism, used to build, repair, and renew body tissues. Since it isn't stored by the body to any great extent, it's needed every single day. The protein you eat is actually broken down into components called amino acids and rebuilt into forms your body can utilize.

The chief source of protein is animal life itself and products thereof: meat, fish, poultry, milk, cheese, eggs. (There are also some vegetable sources: soybeans, nuts, dried peas and beans. And some secondary sources, including whole-wheat breads and cereals—plus a little bit in fruits and vegetables.) We all need protein. It is worth your while to get a pocket calorie counter—not to consult religiously every time you shop for food, but for comparison purposes. All animal products are high in protein. But you will find that ounce for ounce, pork, ham, goose, mackerel, and sausages, for example—all high-protein foods—are also relatively high in calories, ounce for ounce. And that chicken, codfish, sole, beef liver, trout, and sirloin (for example) are, comparatively speaking—while still high in protein—relatively low in calories.

Similarly, the various dairy products that come in different forms differ in calories as well. Whole pasteurized milk is a good source of protein. So is skim milk—which has only the fat, not the protein, removed. Buttermilk, in spite of its name, actually has fewer calories than whole milk. Margarine versus butter? Same number of calories, essentially—but your doctor may recommend the former if there's a hint of high blood cholesterol (which, as you no doubt know, is a suspected culprit in heart disease); margarine, especially the kind made with vegetable oil, does have less saturated fat, which is possibly the prime villain.

Fats are not very necessary in the ordinary diet, certainly something to be avoided if you're aiming at weight loss. The reason is that they are stored in the body—hence, do not need to be resupplied on a daily basis and, though they're needed nutritional components, need not be sought after. They're present in most meats, many fish, all fried foods, all dairy products to a certain extent.

Carbohydrates are the energy foods, the starches and sugars. Again, they're foods we need—but most of us take a lot more of them than our bodies actually require. They, along with fats, are prominent adders of poundage. They include alcoholic beverages and candies and pastries. They are also components of foods that are otherwise beneficial, such as cereals, potatoes, and whole-wheat breads—which offer not mere carbohydrates, but also helpful vitamins and minerals.

Which brings us to *that* subject. You need *not* go out of your way to purchase all sorts of expensive wheat germ cereals, exotic seeds, and mysterious liquid concoctions in order to assure yourself of a balanced, fairly low-calorie diet; the components are all readily available at your local supermarket. If you are doing your shopping with an eye to paring pounds, just select those nutritious items that are relatively low in calories as compared with those that are laden with *both* genuine food values *and* weight-producing calories.

Again, we're not presenting a calorie-counter here. But take vegetables. Fairly high in calories: baked beans, potatoes, lima beans, peas of any kind. Relatively low in calories: greens of any kind, beets, onions, carrots, mushrooms, green beans, asparagus, broccoli, spinach. Similarly, any soups that are creamed and contain a high-calorie vegetable to boot—vichyssoise, other cream soups, and so on—are going to add pounds, while broths and plain poultry or vegetable soups (chicken, onion, vegetable) are less of a threat.

How about vitamins? You certainly need them. You are not likely to have a deficiency of them, unless you are—like many old-time sailors—stranded far out to sea without any fresh citrus fruits on board. Under those circumstances, it is con-

133

ceivable that you might get scurvy, a very nasty disease indeed. If you have no symptoms, you do not have it and are not in danger of getting it. Anyone who has it is acutely conscious of dire symptoms. It can, at any rate, be easily prevented by a landlubber by making sure that you get a daily supply of vitamin C (it is not stored by the body). All citrus fruits contain vitamin C, as do some others, prominently tomatoes, strawberries, and melons.

There are, as not everybody knows, some good vegetable sources of vitamin C as well. These include most green vegetables—spinach, brussels sprouts, etc.—as well as other freshly available items such as cauliflower, potatoes, and sweet potatoes. Other vitamins are clearly essential as well. They are present in every single food we have mentioned. Vitamins A and D are among those with which an overdose is possible if unneeded supplements are taken; they are found especially in fats (liquid or solid) and yellow or leafy vegetables. Vitamin B is derived from both dairy products and whole-grain foods.

Iron, an essential mineral, is found primarily in meats (liver especially), but also in a number of those otherwise beneficial items: poultry, eggs, collards, spinach, other greens. (Vegetablewise a good rule is: dark color=iron.) Other vitamins and minerals are present in small amounts in many foods—and only small amounts are needed; if you concentrate on the major essentials, you'll be getting the minor ones as well.

And what of vitamin E? One of the minor vitamins, first synthesized in 1937, it has been widely promoted over the last several years as having stupendous powers ranging from the dispersal of offensive bodily odors to the prevention of heart disease and the maintenance of sexual prowess, not excluding the relief of such chronic conditions as arthritis. The truth is that only very small amounts are required by the human body, and the principal sources of the B vitamins are excellent sources of vitamin E as well. Lack of vitamin E is not in fact known to cause any detectable illness or disorder. The only recorded cases of vitamin E deficiency perpetrating any sort of inimical condition have involved a particular sort of anemia that has occurred in prematurely born infants, and even then quite uncommonly; it is believed to be related to an absorption disability due to that prematurity. There is *no* evidence that vitamin E deficiency is associated with any arthritic disorder, or that supplementary quantities would be beneficial in the treatment of any such disorder. We suggest that any such "benefits" of which you may have heard are very likely instances of that coincidental spontaneous-remission phenomenon we remarked upon in Chapter 2.

Most of the foods at your local supermarket are reasonably good sources of vitamins, minerals, and other essential food elements. If you're aiming at weight loss, just choose—among the available good sources of nutritional elements—those that are relatively low in calories as opposed to those that are relatively high. It's that simple.

The last sentence is a bit misleading. It is, factually, that simple. One's own eating habits, however, are *not* always quite that amenable to change. It is easy to "resolve" that one will substitute an orange for a potato—but they certainly don't taste the same, and habits are not easily broken. It can, admittedly, be a problem. You're not hugely obese (which requires medical management), just definitely overweight; you want to relieve multiple strains by removing some of those pounds. How do you begin?

Pounds-Paring Hints

The following advice is offered solely within the context of what we have previously said: that a balanced diet must—for your continued health—be maintained, and that your physician must be consulted before adding or subtracting any vital elements or supplements.

With that precaution in mind, here are some simple—and proved workable—hints to help you gradually diminish weight. (It should be noted that weight lost gradually is by and large lost permanently; the more rapid the loss, the faster its reappearance.)

—One thing that often works—it will never make headlines, because it's so very simple—in some who need to lose a fairly small amount is simply to do precisely that: lose small amounts —of portions, of food. Just continue eating everything you normally eat, but shave the portions: take a bowl of cold cereal and put a little back in the box; take one less slice of meat at dinner; when you sugar your coffee, shake a little back into the sugar bowl. If you have been maintaining your weight at a somewhat too high level, and you continue your usual activities, these tricks will effect a gradual weight loss.

—Look for new ways to cook your food that will not add calories. Any frying, for example, does add calories: you're adding fat to whatever you're frying, and some of it is absorbed (no matter what you pour off). Most things that can be fried— hamburger, chops, other red meats, chicken, fish—can also be either broiled or baked, with no added fat.

—When you're attempting gradual weight loss, don't psych yourself out. Meaning, don't weigh yourself daily. Once or twice a week is enough. This kind of little-by-little loss—which

136

is of course the most permanent kind—takes place in such small amounts per day that the readings are likely to discourage you.

–Examine, within the context of whatever you buy. Look for cuts of meat that are less fatty than others, canned fruit that is water- instead of syrup-packed, and the like.

–When you're cooking, be aware of lower-calorie substitutions that can be made in recipes: the various meats and fish, as we mentioned; skim milk for whole milk; lower-calorie for higher-calorie fruits or vegetables. Exercise the same precautions when eating in restaurants.

–When in doubt, zero in on high-protein foods; they satisfy the appetite for a longer period.

–Remember that *hunger* requires *food; habit* demands *particular* foods. Learn to sort them out.

TEN

Sex and Arthritis,
How to Cope with the Question of

This subject has been virtually ignored in other writings on arthritis, perhaps because of various authors' fears of "offending" readers. In physicians' offices, too, the sex lives of arthritis sufferers have often been a taboo subject: in part, we *know*, because patients are reluctant to air their insecurities and fears; in part, we *suspect*, because doctors have been hesitant to broach the topic, to initiate what may seem an invasion of privacy.

A bit of air clearing is unquestionably in order.

Parallel and Paradox

The arthritic disorders are physical ailments. Almost any physical ailment necessitates limitations or restrictions; arthritis (from here on, we'll use this word to encompass any of the arthritic conditions we've talked about in this book, unless otherwise specified) is no exception. But depending upon the nature and prognosis of the problem, one's reactions and attitudes are going to vary a great deal.

Let us take, for example, a broken leg—clearly a physically restrictive condition. Movement is limited. The leg is encased in a cast. One cannot engage in active sports. Simple walking about becomes a strenuous chore. Certainly any physical activities, including sex, will be severely curtailed. But—and this is an important point—the situation is a temporary one; at some point in the near future, conditions will return to normal, with no vestiges (or at least minimal ones) of the limitations lingering on.

Now let's take another example. You find, quite suddenly, that you have developed a severe allergy to chocolate—a substance that has been a continuing, delightful high point in your gustatory spectrum. The doctor advises that, if you are to avoid severe and potentially critical reactions, chocolate must go. If you are ten years of age, this interdiction is likely to prove pretty devastating; not overwhelming, exactly, but it is going to take a lot of getting used to. If, on the other hand, you are sixty years of age, chances are you will realistically shrug your shoulders and find it fairly easy to cross chocolate off your dietary list—simply because by that time, you have encountered a good many other equally enjoyable foods.

Chronic arthritic disorders are, by definition, not specifically limited in duration—quite unlike a fractured leg. That's point one. The course of these disorders is usually unpredictable; while there may be remissions, neither their occurrence nor their duration can be depended upon.

Point two is that sex, unlike the ingestion of chocolate, is not easily dismissed. It is a basic human need—which chocolate is not. To the young, its curtailment could be devastating, particularly during a period when a sexual relationship is just being established. To the older man or woman, accustomed to a thoroughly satisfactory relationship based upon mutually gratifying behavior, a mandated change in that behavior can be—understandably—quite threatening.

Thus the parallels become, in a sense, paradoxical. If you are a young person, still experimenting and exploring and expanding your sexual horizons, unforeseen physical restriction will appear as a barrier, a frustration. If you are older, accustomed to a thoroughly satisfying pattern (call it routine or schedule, if that applies) of sexual performance, arthritic limitations will appear as a threat of waning powers, a sudden catapult "over the hill." In either case, the feeling that will emerge is *insecurity*—individually, and vis-à-vis your sexual partner.

We can say this categorically, because it is a *normal, human* reaction. If you have RA, or OA, or spondylitis, or a number of other conditions we've talked about in earlier chapters, and you have *not* found yourself suffering from some sexual difficulties—or you have been fortunate to have resolved those difficulties with your own spouse or doctor—fine; stop right here. You don't need to read the rest of this chapter. You are a member of the very lucky minority, and/or an extraordinarily resourceful person.

But if you're like most people, the realization that an arthritic condition has put a crimp in your sex life is going to come as rather a blow. You are likely to be frustrated and unhappy, and possibly quite depressed. If you know that's a fact of your life—or of the life of someone you love—then this chapter may give you a new vantage point.

Start with the Status Quo

Some of what follows is going to be very obvious to some readers, eye-opening to others. The explanation of that statement lies in the realm of the psychological.

When we are faced with medical facts, we have varying

reactions, depending upon our differing personalities. We may exaggerate them, seeing them as worse than they are. We may accept them at face value, but ignore their ramifications. We may dismiss them because we choose to believe they do not exist. Or—hopefully—we may accept them, consider them, and view them anew in the light of their broader implications.

Obviously, we are urging the last option. Sexual intercourse is a physical activity. If the way you have been engaging in that activity is now uncomfortable or painful or even—because, say, of limited joint movement—impossible, that's just not the end of the world, however it may appear. Plenty of other activities must, in fact, be forgone because of arthritis: a particular arthritic condition may preclude tennis, or bowling, or mountain climbing. But *not* sex—not if your mind is open.

Let's spell it out. Tennis, bowling, or mountain climbing demands use of certain joints: wrists, knees, elbows, ankles. If you are right-handed, and your arthritis afflicts your right elbow, you will probably accept some temporary or permanent modification of your tennis game. No bowler is going to function well without full, flexible use of hip and knee joints. Mountain climbing is a challenge to the individual with all skeletal and muscular structures in optimum condition. Sexual intercourse? Neither the male's equipment—penis, testes—nor the female's—vagina and external appurtenances—are remotely subject to arthritic disorders. Whether you have OA, RA, spondylitis, or any other arthritic problem, it does *not* affect your capacity for enjoyment of sexual relations. Not directly.

What *may* be affected are the mechanics of achieving that sexual gratification, and that's the crux of the question. There is also a secondary difficulty; it might be well to consider it first, since it's often more easily resolved.

That factor is simple fatigue. Most couples have sexual relations in late evening, at the end of the day's other activities.

Sex and Arthritis

Fatigue may ensue under the most ideal circumstances; arthritis is apt to increase that fatigue. Exhaustion coupled with taut, aching muscles is not conducive to eagerness for energetic sex play. But there are, in fact, some practical answers to the dilemma. Any one or more of the following may be helpful.

–Try lying back in a hot bath for as long as an hour before engaging in sexual relations; you'll find it wonderfully relaxing for tense, knotted muscles—and a good antidote for emotional tensions, too.

–Discuss with your doctor the possibility of prescribing a muscle-relaxant medication that also acts as a mild "tranquilizer"; diazepam (Valium), chlordiazepoxide (Librium), and oxazepam (Serax)—all of which belong to a class of therapeutic agents called benzodiazepines—are among those that many people find particularly effective. A small dose taken about an hour before planned sexual relations can prove an effective easer of both mental and physical tensions.

–Contemplate a change of schedule, so far as your sex life goes. Sure, most people do find evenings most convenient. But there's no prohibition applying to other times of day. Depending upon your particular arthritic condition, it might work out better first thing in the morning, for example (although in rheumatoid arthritis, early-morning stiffness may preclude that solution). Or if a husband's job is near home, near enough to come home for lunch, and his wife's home during the day, and the kids are off at school, that may prove a workable solution.

Some Pertinent Principles

Speaking of drugs, which we have alluded to very briefly, there are some that are *not* likely to enhance sexual enjoyment —in fact, just the opposite. It is good to be aware of them. Alcohol, for example, is likely to increase sexual desire—but decrease male ability to perform; the same is true of ampheta-mines. Also, certain powerful (narcotic) analgesics that are sometimes prescribed for serious pain, often to be taken at bed-time—among such drugs are Demerol and Percodan—will dampen desire for sexual relations.

A few other basic physiological and psychological factors might be relevant at this point, factors not restricted to the problems peculiar to arthritis (to which we shall return shortly).

One of these is that the human male needs—*physically* needs—periodic spermatic release. That need may be affected by other ills, but it is not changed by arthritis. It increases with lapse of time. Thus, longer intervals between sexual relations often mean that release may be achieved more quickly and easily.

Another is that sensory tolerance develops with continued, unvaried sensory input—sexual or other. Distracting noise—say, in a work situation—can irritate at first, but many studies have shown that as it continues at the same level, it can success-fully be screened out; it is not reacted to, and for all practical purposes is not "heard." Similarly with any kind of stimuli, in-cluding sexual. When sexual relations become stereotyped, unvarying, mechanical, they are no longer stimulating.

It is a truism that the prospect of enjoyable sexual relations is enhanced if each partner makes an effort to appeal to the other—not only emotionally or verbally, but physically as well. The housewife with rheumatoid arthritis who has been through a tiring day hopes that sexual relations with her husband at the end of that day will be a leisurely, pleasant, relaxing affair. If he makes a habit of arriving home sweaty and grimy from the the body-and-fender shop, and without pausing for a bath or shower or any other preliminary niceties, insists upon instant retirement for a fast fling in the bedroom—well, she is going to feel less than enthusiastic; her fatigue and depression are going to loom very large, and said husband should not be surprised if he receives a flat "No, I'm too tired, and it's been an especially bad day!" There are going to be a lot of bad days.

Of course there are two sides to that coin. A man with spondylitis, whose sheer physical disability makes intercourse difficult, is not going to be glowing with eager self-confidence if the object of his affections presents herself attired in her least attractive housecleaning costume, hair in curlers, sticky cream all over her face, and dirt under her fingernails.

In short, your making an effort to appeal to your partner sexually means that you are interested, that your partner is desirable, that he or she is not being taken for granted.

Before we come to some specific suggestions, there are a couple of other basic facts of which you should be aware. They *are* facts, despite the continuing proliferation of rumors and old wives' tales. It is difficult to rid oneself of superstitions and mistaken ideas that may have been deeply ingrained in childhood and early adulthood.

One is that sexual activity, once initiated, must lead inevitably and invariably to orgasm. It need not. If you and your partner enjoy activities of whatever kind or degree, from simple fondling to manual-genital stimulation, and you do not care to continue to orgasmic climax on that occasion, there is no rule that obliges you to do so. What is foreplay on one occasion may well be the whole game on another.

A second concept we urge you to discard is that sexual intercourse must always be performed in particular body positions. Fish, terriers, and ostriches do indeed carry on their sexual relations by ritual instinct. Human beings need not. Human beings have imagination and the capacity for creative thought, and can devise and learn new and alternate means of achieving desired goals. We'll have more to say about that.

The third insidiously pervasive superstition concerns masturbation. Generations of parents have now accepted the idea, via simple observation, that infants and small children are likely to start to masturbate, and to continue doing so quite frequently, as soon as they make the discovery that fingering their genitals provides a pleasant sensation. Many of those individuals, grown to adulthood, feel somehow that masturbation is shameful. Some of them have even gotten the mistaken notion that masturbation can and will precipitate a host of dire conditions ranging from acne to impotence, from mental degeneration to outright insanity. None of these things are true.

Masturbation is, in short, a universal practice and not a symptom of any sort of derangement.

Practical Matters

Let us assume, now, that you and your partner have previously enjoyed a stimulating and satisfying sexual relationship. And now, that relationship is suffering. Perhaps because what was pleasurable before has become painful; perhaps because a once-supple joint has become inflexible; perhaps because a limb that would once bear weight now falters.

Because each human being, and each case of arthritis, and each sexual relationship are unique, we cannot prescribe solutions for your individual problems. Your challenge, in effect, is to find new ways of engaging in sexual relations—ways that will continue to afford you pleasure and will circumvent or minimize the present physical problem. What follows, then, are simply a few examples—ideas that we hope will help you, perhaps in consultation with your own physician or with a sympathetic counselor specializing in the improvement of sexual relations, to arrive at the answers that will be right for *you*.

Some Examples of Problems	*Some Possible Solutions*
Spondylitis—in which endurance is a frequent difficulty.	Extensive manual foreplay, permitting less strenuous effort on the male partner's part. Also, as previously noted, less frequent activity—which hastens release when sexual relations do take place.
Scleroderma, often involving respiratory difficulty, even without strenuous activity.	Let that individual play the most passive role and assume the most passive position, to minimize fatiguing physical activity.
Hips, with pain on flexing—i.e., bending the thighs toward the torso—in a woman with rheumatoid arthritis.	Supine (on her back) position, with her legs straight, perhaps a pillow beneath the hips.
Knees with pain on bending.	Wear knee guards for support and for preventing flexion—and choose positions that put no weight on the knees. A woman with this problem can choose to use a chaise longue, her partner seated while she sits on his lap (facing him or not) with pillows at either side supporting her legs. A man with afflicted knees might choose the supine position, while his partner sits astride him.

Some Examples of Problems	*Some Possible Solutions*
One afflicted hip or knee.	Lateral — on-the-side — positions for both partners, with the afflicted side upward to avoid all pressure on it (the woman can face her partner or away from him).
A single joint that's chronically painful, pain that proves unbearably distracting.	A short-term "anesthetic" in the form of a cold pack applied to that joint just before.
Afflicted knees that become painful upon close bodily embrace.	Avoid intertwining the legs. It is pressure above the knee—i.e., around the thigh—that often precipitates the pain.
All-over achiness, when just about any activity hurts.	Achieve climax via mutual manual means.

As we've said, these are simply a few examples, with a few possible solutions. What's needed is, basically, common sense. Observe what movements, what positions are exacerbating the problem—and look for alternates. Aside from oral and manual activities, realize that it is possible for a man and woman to have sexual intercourse on practically any kind of furniture; lying down (with either partner underneath), sitting, kneeling, or standing; with the female facing her partner or with her back to him. No one way is "right" and none are "wrong." The way or ways that are right for you are those that give you pleasure and do not cause you pain.

The Bottom Line

Perhaps it's obvious, but we'll say it anyway. All that we have been discussing in this chapter, the attainment (or reattainment) of good and satisfying relations between the arthritic patient and his or her sexual partner, demands one vital factor at the start: complete honesty and frankness between the partners. The patient should not play martyr, but should fully explain his or her feelings and discomforts, pains and pleasures —and insecurities, too. The partner (who, we hope, will have read the preceding chapters and so gained an understanding of the illness itself) must develop understanding and sympathy, adapt to the afflicted partner's limitations—and, above all, actively cooperate in seeking solutions that will be satisfying to both.

Many a physician can affirm that often, when food restrictions have been imposed upon a patient, the exercise of creative imagination has actually resulted in the new diet's being more interesting and enjoyable than the old. That can apply, and has applied, in the area of sexual relations as well.

ELEVEN

Just Around the Corner:
Hints Emerge from Research

In a number of earlier chapters, we noted some of the more intriguing questions that have been and are being raised about the causes and treatments of the various arthritic disorders. Here, we single out a few areas of recent investigation and theory that may, in time, lead to surer and more effective therapies. Some are even now being studied in laboratory or clinic. Others exist solely in the realm of speculation. None can be dismissed in the continuing quest for control of this baffling group of ills.

Acupuncture

As the reader must be aware, there has been intense Western interest in this ancient Oriental technique ever since the first American scientists visited mainland China and returned with their newsmaking reports in 1971. Newspaper headlines, in the main, have played up the use of the needles for surgical anesthesia—a use that has been hailed as miraculous in some quarters, condemned as outright fakery in others. Acupuncture anesthesia—whether valid in itself or, as some feel, useful only when backed by sedatives or hypnosis—is in fact a fairly new idea, even in China; it has been in use only since the late 1950s. Far more venerable is the use of acupuncture as analgesia, for the relief of chronic pain, and it is of course that possibility that holds special interest for arthritics.

A number of reports from Europe, where acupuncture has been used more widely than in our country, have suggested that the technique may be useful in the relief of fairly mild pain such as that of early rheumatoid arthritis and osteoarthritis; one physician, in France, has also reported finding it effective in diminishing the pangs of acute gout in some patients. At this writing, an extensive and intensive study has been launched by the National Institutes of Health, and experts in anesthesiology, neurology, and psychology are evaluating the technique and its overall potentials for use in American medicine.

Individual physicians on this side of the Atlantic, particularly those with a special knowledge of acupuncture, have also been looking into its potential for pain relief. Dr. James Y. P. Chen of the California Medical Group in Los Angeles reported to a government-sponsored research conference early in 1973 that he had found acupuncture effective in some 70 percent of a group of patients suffering from various types of chronic pain (just over a quarter of the group were victims of osteoarthritis). Dr. Teruo Matsamoto of Philadelphia also reported good results in a small group of osteoarthritis patients.

As we pointed out in an early chapter, definitive evaluation of therapeutic techniques—whether medications or other procedures—properly requires careful comparisons; such techniques must be weighed against other, known therapies, as well as against nontreatment (especially vital in arthritis, with its well-known spontaneous-remission patterns).

A controlled study in rheumatoid arthritis patients conducted by Dr. C. S. Man of the University of Manitoba in

Canada, who has been schooled in both Oriental and Western medicine, sought to evaluate the comparative effects of steroid injection and acupuncture, as well as any psychological "suggestion" element that might be present. All the patients in the study suffered from continuing knee pain. For a number of months, one knee of each patient received periodic injections of corticosteroids, while the other was treated by acupuncture —but with a slight "twist": a third variable, unknown to the patients, was introduced. Half the patients received their acupuncture in the traditionally "correct" manner, while in the others, the needles were deliberately mis-inserted—i.e., at sites not in accord with the prescribed technique for relief of knee pain. In effect, half the patients thus received a "placebo" —an apparent treatment that was not really a treatment—in one knee. Throughout the study, discomfort during various activities was gauged, the need for additional pain-relieving medications was recorded, and objective evidence was obtained via signs of inflammatory activity such as swelling and heat emission.

The results of Dr. Man's study, reported in June 1973 to a meeting of the American Rheumatism Association section of the Arthritis Foundation, were quite interesting. "Placebo" acupuncture, as expected, proved statistically ineffectual (10 percent of the patients so treated reported some relief of pain —which might, of course, have occurred without any ministrations at all). Steroids, also as expected, were clearly effective in reducing both pain (in 80 percent) and local heat and swelling (in 50 percent). But acupuncture (that is, the *real* acupuncture treatment), while it reduced swelling in only 10 percent and had no measurable effect whatever on heat, actually outperformed steroids in pain relief, with a 90 percent achievement record; the duration of relief with acupuncture (one to three months) also proved longer than that achieved with steroids (two to six weeks). The ideal interval for acupuncture treatment for pain relief, Dr. Man estimated, might range from every three to six months in mild RA to weekly in very severe cases.

A number of other rheumatologists, including several whose research is being supported by the Arthritis Foundation, are also conducting controlled studies. Meanwhile, the foundation has warned, arthritis patients seeking pain relief should be wary of rushing to the nearest self-proclaimed acupuncture "expert." Many such individuals are basically quacks seeking, as charlatans have done for centuries, to capitalize on the credulity of those seeking surcease from chronic pain. Thorough and painstaking investigations are needed before acupuncture —or any untried technique—can be judged truly effective.

There is also the question of the legal status of acupuncture and its practitioners. Various states have promulgated regulations, ranging from broadly permissive to stringently restrictive. In Nevada, for example, the legislature decided acupuncturists need not even be physicians; the New York State Board of Medicine, on the other hand, concluded that, pending further study, acupuncture may be practiced only by, or under the supervision of, licensed physicians, and only in medical schools, teaching hospitals, or other properly qualified medical research institutions; and the state of Kansas outlawed it completely.

Federal attitudes will, in any case, probably take precedence over any positions adopted by individual states. Dr. Joseph B. Davis, director of the Division of Scientific Review of the Food and Drug Administration's Office of Medical Services, has warned at this writing that acupuncture is viewed strictly as a matter for research, and is not approved for general use. Dr. Davis notes that arthritis patients in particular, especially if they are in severe pain, may be, and we quote, "gullible victims for the so-called acupuncture clinics run by medical practitioners of dubious expertise and medical ability. Some of them are less concerned about establishing the safety and efficacy of acupuncture as a possible valuable adjunct to the practice of medicine than they are about the patient's pocketbook."

Finally, this comment. Whatever the potential acupuncture offers for pain relief, it is certainly not a *cure*. As the Arthritis Foundation has succinctly noted: "Chairman Mao Tse-Tung is reputed to be crippled by arthritis. It is reasonable to assume that he has undergone acupuncture treatment performed by the best available specialists, and yet he sometimes can hardly walk."

Drugs New and Old

None of the anti-inflammatory medications is without its risks; even aspirin, certainly the safest, brings with it in large doses and prolonged use the threat of serious side effects. Thus, there is a constant search for new formulations, for drugs that will effectively halt inflammation and its accompanying pain and at the same time present minimal risks or hazards.

Among those under study at this writing—and there are quite a few—one called benorylate, which is being tested in Europe, seems particularly promising. Chemically related to aspirin, it has appeared in early trials to be as effective as aspirin but possibly less likely to give rise to the secondary, unwanted effects that have been noted with aspirin.

A second drug, which has been under investigation in our own country for several years (the senior author has already participated in one published study), is a medication called ibuprofen (Motrin); it may well emerge as a valuable alternative to aspirin for victims of rheumatoid arthritis who have evidenced sensitivity or other untoward reactions to aspirin. The drug seems unusually effective in diminishing morning stiffness, about equivalent to aspirin in most other benefits. Significantly fewer undesirable reactions have been reported in the various trials, however, especially gastrointestinal intolerance—evidenced by nausea, vomiting, stomach pain, diarrhea or constipation—and other known side effects of long-term aspirin therapy, such as dizziness or ringing in the ears. Further clinical investigation of ibuprofen continues, in an effort to establish dosages that will achieve optimal balance between good and ill effects.

Two other agents should perhaps be noted—not because they appear to offer any great potential, but because the reader may have seen enthusiasm about them expressed elsewhere.

One is mefenamic acid, a minor analgesic unrelated to the salicylates. Thus far there is no evidence that it is superior to aspirin, and there has been mounting evidence of far more perilous side effects, including gastrointestinal disturbances, neurological reactions, and anemia. The other is dimethyl sulfoxide (DMSO), a substance applied topically (on the skin) rather than taken internally; although it appears to have some analgesic properties, there are indications that it may cause serious blood abnormalities, and it has not been approved in this country for other than experimental use.

Sometimes it is found that drugs designed to deal with one sort of condition may be effective for another. Thus, in addition to seeking and evaluating brand-new substances, researchers frequently review the existing pharmacopoeia to see if medications already available might be useful in other situations.

One such drug is penicillamine, a "relative" of penicillin that is a specific for the treatment of lead poisoning and for a hereditary condition called Wilson's disease in which there is a disturbance in the body's handling of copper. In early 1973, the results of a British study using this drug for severe, advanced rheumatoid arthritis were announced.

All of the 105 patients in the study had failed to respond to conventional, accepted treatment—aspirin, other anti-inflammatory drugs, gold salts, and so on. The study was double-blind; that is, each patient was randomly assigned to receive penicillamine or a placebo, and neither patients nor physicians knew which substance was being taken. There was, as expected, no improvement in the fifty-three patients receiving the placebo; nine of them, in fact, had to be dropped from the study because their condition worsened. The fifty-two subjects receiving penicillamine showed definite improvement: there was diminution of pain and morning stiffness, decreased inflammation, and a generally heightened feeling of well-being; none got worse during the course of treatment. As with many potent drugs, however, there are side effects, and sixteen of the fifty-two taking penicillamine (31 percent) were dropped from the study because of such effects; the side effects include rash, kidney malfunction, gastrointestinal discomfort, internal bleeding, and loss of the sense of taste.

Penicillamine is now approved for the treatment of severe RA in Great Britain, but has *not* at this writing been so approved in the United States. Further studies are measuring its efficacy as compared with gold salts and other potent medications, as well as exploring its possible use in decreased dosages in early, less severe RA.

Hormones?

Chiefly because of the apparent preference of some of the arthritic disorders for one sex or the other—as well as the frequent improvement of rheumatoid arthritis during pregnancy —there has been recurrent speculation on the role that hormones in general, and the sex hormones in particular, may play. Generally, such speculations have led nowhere. One recent

Swiss study did demonstrate some success in treating scleroderma (PSS) with progestogens, agents similar to an ovarian
hormone; 90 percent of the patients in the study, in fact,
seemed to benefit. Substantial improvement, however, was
limited to skin involvement; effects on arthritic and other
symptoms were minimal.

Blood Flow and Biofeedback

It's possible that sufferers from rheumatoid arthritis could
benefit by borrowing from research in another ailment, migraine headache.

There is a recently developed diagnostic technique called
thermography, by which differentials in skin temperature can
be measured and depicted graphically. What is measured is
surface heat; the major factor in the body's emission of surface
heat is the blood flow to the area involved. It has been determined, via thermography, that the hands of some migraine
patients are abnormally cold—and that increasing blood flow
to the hands and thus warming them, while at the same time
cooling the head, can provide a measure of relief from head
pain.

That finding has led one group of investigators to a unique
approach: the use of a very new technique called biofeedback.
The term "feedback" comes from electronics and means a return or "backflow" of information or signals to the original
source; the "bio" prefix is from the Greek *bios*, "life." Thus,
the biofeedback concept suggests that an individual, observing
continuous readings of information about his own body, might
use that knowledge to actually affect and alter those readings.
In the experimental studies with the migraine patients, temperature sensors are placed on the head and hands, and the

patient can observe the temperature differentials on a meter. It has been found that some patients, after intensive training and practice—especially involving relaxing techniques—can gradually learn to control the meter readings by somehow "making" their heads cooler and their hands warmer. The object, of course, is to abandon the sensors and meters eventually and to master the technique so that it can be used at will anywhere, at any time. Some cannot learn to do so. Many others, of course, simply do not have the patience to go through the training. But those who have succeeded have experienced gratifying relief from their headaches.

The connection with rheumatoid arthritis? Just this: in some RA patients, too, thermography has revealed alterations in blood flow to the extremities—to the fingers, and to the toes as well. Although the biofeedback technique has not yet, to our knowledge, been applied to RA, such an approach may be well worth a trial in those patients in whom the temperature differentials have been demonstrated.

Histidine

Histidine is an amino acid found normally in human serum; levels of this substance are unusually low in RA patients. While the significance of this phenomenon is unknown, it has been postulated that perhaps administration of the substance would have some salutary effect on the course of the disease.

There have been several investigations, none as yet conclusive. The latest, reported early in 1973, was a double-blind study conducted jointly by Dartmouth and the State University of New York. As with the penicillamine project we detailed earlier, half the patients received the substance under study, the others an inert placebo. The results were a bit puzzling. In the placebo group, those patients with fairly mild disease and low erythrocyte sedimentation rates (see page 81) actually improved! But in the histidine group, it was those patients who had more severe arthritis of longer duration, a greater degree of functional impairment, positive tests for the rheumatoid factor (see page 81), and higher sed rates, who showed improvement—not great improvement, but improvement nonetheless.

Certainly further studies (this was the first double-blind one) are needed before this substance can be considered a significant RA therapy, even for a small subgroup of patients. Histidine needs to be compared with other, accepted therapies such as aspirin, gold salts, indomethacin, and the butazones. Various dosage levels need to be tried (the first trials of L-dopa, the drug now known to be effective for Parkinsonism, were thought to prove the therapy useless—until later studies showed that the earlier doses had simply been too small). Larger, longer studies are called for (the Dartmouth-SUNY study involved only sixty patients and lasted only thirty days). And it would certainly be helpful to find out what the low histidine levels in RA patients signify in the first place—and whether they are a cause or a result of the basic disorder.

Cyclic AMP and the Prostaglandins

These terms may be unfamiliar to some of our readers. But it is certain that you will be hearing more and more about them. Perhaps by the time you read this, certainly within the next few years, they are likely to have become "household words."

AMP stands for adenosine monophosphate; the "cyclic" refers not to time periods but to a characteristic of its molecular structure. Isolated in 1958 by Dr. Earl Sutherland, Jr., a distinguished physiologist (he received a Nobel Prize in 1971), cyclic AMP proved to be a sort of "missing link" in our knowledge of the biochemical processes of the body. Dr. Sutherland dubbed it a "second messenger"; his description is an apt one. While various hormones produced by the endocrine glands have long been known to influence and regulate functions and processes in many parts of the body, it now appears that they do not do so directly: rather, it is cyclic AMP that "relays" the hormone's "message."

But this chemical plays other roles as well. Subsequent research has shown that among other things it stimulates the release of certain hormones, plays a role in regulating fat metabolism, inhibits the growth of certain tumor cells, and triggers the actions of a number of enzymes in the liver and elsewhere; animal experiments suggest that abnormally low levels in blood vessels may contribute to high blood pressure. The list of its actions and probable actions is in fact virtually endless, as are its clinical possibilities.

Certainly it seems to hold the hope of being a major cancer fighter; it has already been shown to act not only against cultured tumor cells, but against actual tumors in laboratory animals. Measurements of cyclic-AMP levels in patients with a number of disorders suggest that it may play a part in therapy for some glandular and kidney dysfunctions. Bronchial asthma and myasthenia gravis, a serious neuromuscular disorder, may involve a disturbance in cyclic-AMP activity. And it may have a therapeutic part to play in the arthritic disorders as well; one research project has already shown that the inflammation of induced arthritis in dogs in the laboratory can be reduced by the injection of cyclic AMP.

Cyclic AMP also is known to react to the prostaglandins—which brings us to that subject.

Contrary to most medical terminology, which is typically very precise and definitive, the word *prostaglandin* is actually a total misnomer. These substances were first discovered in the early 1930s in seminal fluids, and it was concluded that they originated in the prostate gland—hence the obvious coining of the name. We now know that there are many of these substances—fourteen have been definitely pinpointed at this writing—and they are actually formed and found in just about all parts of the body, from the skin to all the vital organs, and including the joints. As more and more data have emerged concerning their functions and actions, it has become clear that the prostaglandins represent one of the most exciting and promising frontiers in twentieth-century medicine.

What is especially fascinating is that some of the identified prostaglandins behave in ways contradictory to some of the others—suggesting that activity by one that causes some disorder, for example, might be successfully countered by the administration of another. A look at some of those activities will give you an idea of the vast possibilities.

As they have been identified, the various prostaglandins have been given distinguishing letters (PGA, PGB, and so on) according to their chemical structures; further variations have been indicated by subscripted numbers, sometimes by Greek-letter suffixes. Here, for instance, are some of the actions of the prostaglandins that have been documented:

–Several of the PGAs and PGEs are vasodilators (dilators of blood vessels); they can produce facial flushing and severe headache.

–PGA_2 and PGE_2 are both present in the renal medulla, a part of the kidney, and may play major roles in regulating blood pressure. Both PGA_1 and PGA_2 can in fact lower blood pressure, and it is further suspected that some antihypertensive drugs work by promoting PGE_2 formation. PGF_2-alpha, on the other hand, is a vasoconstrictor, and also *raises* blood pressure.

–The PGEs can effectively counter such conditions as peptic ulcer (by inhibiting gastric secretions), asthma (by relaxing bronchial spasms), nasal congestion, and a variety of allergic reactions.

–PGE_1 has been found in laboratory animals to reduce the inflammation of experimentally induced arthritis, apparently by stabilizing lysosomal membranes (see pages 7–8). PGE_2 and PGF_2-alpha, though, apparently play active roles in *creating* inflammation; anti-inflammatory agents such as aspirin, indomethacin, and the corticosteroids act, at least in part, by attacking a precursor substance called arachidonic acid, thus preventing prostaglandin formation.

–PGE_2 is the chief prostaglandin synthesized in human skin; it is formed notably faster following a wound or burn, and it is known to encourage blood clotting. Yet in victims of sickle-cell disease, PGE_2 has been found to increase the production of the abnormally distorted red blood cells (obviously, an anti-PGE_2 agent might prove very helpful for victims of this hereditary anemia).

–Both PGE_2 and PGF_2-alpha have the property of stimulating uterine contractions in pregnant women. PGF_2-alpha also drastically reduces the secretion of a hormone needed to insure implantation of a fertilized egg cell in the uterus; thus it might one day play a role in "morning-after" contraception.

–PGE_1 acts on many different tissues and organs, including the thyroid, the lungs, and the spleen, to increase levels of cyclic AMP. But in combination with epinephrine or ACTH, it acts on fat tissue to *decrease* cyclic AMP—as do PGA_1, PGE_2, and PGF_1-alpha. PGE_1 and PGE_2, acting together, effect an increased level of cyclic AMP in platelets, the "clotting cells" of the blood.

None of the prostaglandins are yet available for clinical use in the United States, and none are likely to be before 1975 or 1976. In late 1972, however, two of them—PGE_2 and PGF_2-alpha, trade-named Prostin E_2 and Prostin F_2-alpha—became commercially available in Great Britain, marketed by a pharmaceutical firm known to have been investigating the synthesis of the substances from certain chemicals found in sea corals. Both these prostaglandins have been promoted chiefly for the purpose of inducing abortion or labor, and were originally available only for administration by injection; they were said to be soon available in oral form.

Obviously the PGEs, and PGE_1 in particular, would seem to have the highest potential for therapeutic use in the arthritic disorders, among those prostaglandins that have been identified to date. For the sake of completeness, however, it must be added that although PGE_1 has been found effective in combating arthritis in laboratory animals, the animals did develop temporary side effects, including diarrhea, hair loss, and inordinate drowsiness. Of course it is not yet known whether or not human arthritis sufferers will evidence the same responses, favorable or otherwise.

INDEX

Acetaminophen, 59, 104
Acetohexamide, interaction with gout medications, 59–60
Acetylsalicylic acid. See Aspirin
ACTH, 55, 115
Acupuncture, 151–55
Acute attack: exercise vs. rest in, 119–20; in gout, 49, 53–56; prevention, 120; in rheumatoid arthritis, 83–84, 85, 90; in spondylitis, 95
Addictive drugs, 109–11
Adenosine monophosphate, 160–62
Adrenal hormones. See Corticosteroids
Advertising, drug, xi, xii, 17–19, 61, 103, 104
Age of victims: of arthritic disorders generally, xi, xiv–xv; of dermatomyositis, 39; of gout, 50; of osteoarthritis, 64, 66, 68–69, 70, of rheumatoid arthritis, 80, 90–91; of scleroderma, 41; of spondylitis, 94; of systemic lupus erythematosus, 26–27
Alcohol: danger of combining with medications, 34, 38, 59, 100, 110, 111; and gout attack, 47, 49, 52; and scleroderma, 42; and sexual relations, 143–44
Alka-Seltzer, 105
Allergy: as factor in rheumatic fever, 31; to medications, 58, 86, 105–6, 107, 108, 110; in mistaken diagnosis, 92; theory in two

arthritic diseases, 30–31, 82
Allopurinol, 57–58, 60–61
American Board of Internal Medicine, 5
American Medical Association (AMA), 21, 119
American Pharmaceutical Association, 103
American Rheumatism Association, xiii, 5, 28, 90, 153
Anacin, 103
Analgesics: abuse of, 102, 109; combined with tranquilizers or sedatives, 111; interactions with other drugs, 34, 38, 59, 60, 100; over-the-counter, 102–6; prescription, 106–10; and sexual relations, 144
Anemia: as effect of medication, 86, 104; associated with two arthritic diseases, 28, 81
Animal diseases resembling human arthritis, 30, 83
Ankylosing spondylitis. See Spondylitis
Antacids, 104–5; interaction with other medications, 34, 101
Antibiotics: interaction with probenecid, 59; useless as therapy, 82–83
Antibodies: action of, 7, 29; antinuclear, test for, 93; medications countering, 36
Anticholesterol drugs, interaction with aspirin, 100–1

165

Index

Hormones. *See* ACTH; Corticosteroids; Sex hormones
Housework, 77, 125–28
Humidity, 124–25
"Humors" theory of illness, 2, 14, 45–46
Hydralazine, 31
Hydroxychloroquine, 34
Hypersensitivity. *See* Allergy
Hypertension: contraindications in, 108; and corticosteroids, 113; medication for, as cause of arthritic disease, 31; and prognosis in scleroderma, 42
Hyperuricemia, 47–48, 51, 61–62
Hypoglycemics. *See* Diabetes

Ibuprofen, 155–56
Immunosuppressives, Imuran (azathioprine), 35–38; interaction with allopurinol, 60
Incidence: of arthritic disorders, *xi*; of collagen diseases, 25; of gout, 50; of osteoarthritis, 64, 66; of psoriatic arthritis, 79; of rheumatoid arthritis, 79; of spondylitis, 79, 94; of systemic lupus erythematosus, 26, 31–32. *See also* Age; Sex
Indocin (indomethacin), 107–8; interaction with aspirin, 101; and prostaglandins, 163
Infection: arthritis associated with systemic, 3–4; fungal, 114; localized in joint, 74, 92; masked by medication, 113; as possible cause of arthritic disorders, 4, 29–30, 42, 82–83, 91, 92; as precursor of osteoarthritis, 69; susceptibility increased in certain therapies, 35–36
Inflammation, 6–7; atypical in osteoarthritis, 73, 74; classic picture of, in gout 49; damage caused by, 118; drugs to combat, *see* Anti-inflammatories; effect in rheumatoid arthritis, 80–81; exacerbated by exercise, 119–20
Injury: as cause of arthritis, 3; and diagnosis in children, 92; and gout attack, 49; healing slowed by drugs, 113; as precursor of osteoarthritis, 69, 70; susceptibility to, 120–21
Insulin, effects and interactions with arthritic medications: butazones, 109; corticosteroids, 114; immunosuppressives, 38; sulfinpyrazone, 60
Interactions of drugs, 100–1. *See also* specific medications. Major interactions are included in discussions of drugs used for arthritic disorders; many used for other conditions, with which such interactions may occur, are indexed separately.
Iridocyclitis, 93
Iron supplements in combination with allopurinol, 60–61

Jaundice, 88
Joint disease as precursor of osteoarthritis, 69
Joint replacement surgery, 74–75, 89
Joints typically affected: in gout, 48; in osteoarthritis, 67, 69–71; in pseudogout, 62; in rheumatoid arthritis, 80; in spondylitis, 94
Journal of the American Medical Association, 119
Juvenile rheumatoid arthritis, 90–93

Kenacort, 112
Kindeys: affected in systemic lupus erythematosus, 28, 31; damaged by certain drugs, 104; disease of, and secondary gout, 61–62; dysfunction of, and containdications,

Index

Posture, role of: in osteoarthritis, 70, 76; in spondylitis, 94, 95, 96, 122
Potentiation (defined), 100
Prednisolone, Prednisone. See Corticosteroids
Pregnancy: contraindications in, 107, 109; drug risks in, 101, 114; and rheumatoid arthritis, 84
Prescriptions, patient's knowledge of, 37, 97–99
Probenecid, 56–60, 103
Procainamide, 31
Prognoses. See specific conditions
Progressive systemic sclerosis (PSS), 41–43, 147
Pronestyl (procainamide), 31
Propoxyphene, 109–10
Prostaglandins, 162–64
Protein. See Nutrition
Pseudogout, 62; diagnosis vs. osteoarthritis, 74
Psoriasis: arthritis in, see Rheumatoid arthritis (diagnostic difference, 81–82); and chloroquines, 85; lesions vs. dermatomyositis, 39; and methotrexate, 85
PSS, 41–43, 147
Psychotherapy, 90
Public Health Service, U. S., 117
Puffiness: in dermatomyositis, 40; in reaction to drugs, 109, 113; in scleroderma, 42
Purines, 47, 52

Quacks, 16, 20–24, 154–55
Quinacrine, 34
Quinine derivatives, 34, 85

RA. See Rheumatoid arthritis
Rash: in reaction to medication, 58, 88, 106, 108, 110; as symptom, 27, 28, 90
Referred pain: in children, 92; in osteoarthritis, 71–72; in spondylitis, 94–95

Relaxants. See Tranquilizers
Relaxation. See Rest
Remission, spontaneous, 23; in rheumatoid arthritis, 83, 84, 91; in spondylitis, 94, 95; in systemic lupus erythematosus, 28
Research: on future therapies, 151–64; methods, 23; money expended for, xiii-xiv, 40. See also specific disorders
Rest, importance of, 92, 96, 119–20. See also Fatigue
Rheumatic diseases (defined), 4–5.
Rheumatic fever, 3, 31, 92
"Rheumatism," 5, 63
Rheumatoid arthritis (RA), 79–90, 106, 108, 110, 147; and caffeine, 103–4; juvenile, 90–93; vs. osteoarthritis, 72; vs. pseudogout, form of, 62; vs. scleroderma, 42; vs. systemic lupus erythematosus, 27. See also Research
Rheumatoid factor, 81–82, 91
Rheumatoid spondylitis. See Spondylitis
Rheumatologist (defined), 5
Rita, Giuseppe, 50
Robert B. Brigham Hospital, 90
Rubella: arthritis associated with, 3, 23; vaccination, 92–93
Rufus of Ephesus, 45

Salicylamide, 104
Salicylates 102–6; interaction with uricosurics, 59, 60. See also Aspirin
Scheinfeld, Amram, 32n
Scleroderma (PSS), 41–43, 147
Secondary gout, 61–62
Sed rate, 81, 88, 95
Sedatives, 110–11; abuse of, 102; interaction with alcohol and other drugs, 38, 59, 100
Self-limited arthritis, 23, 41
Serax (oxazepam), 95–96, 110–11, 143

Index

Symptoms: in dermatomyositis, 39–40; in gout, 48–49; in osteoarthritis, 65, 67–68, 71–73; in rheumatoid arthritis, 80, 90–91; in scleroderma, 41–42; in spondylitis, 93–95; in systemic lupus erythematosus, 27–28
Synergism (defined), 100
Synovectomy, 88–89
Synovial membrane, 48, 62, 73, 88–89, 119–20
Synovitis (defined), 62
Systemic lupus erythematosus (SLE), 26–38, 92

Talwin (pentazocine), 109–10
Tandearil (oxyphenbutazone), 108–9; contraindicated in children, 92
Temperature, effects of, 84, 124–25. *See also* Cold; Heat
Tempra (acetaminophen), 59, 104
Tendons, 5, 28, 48, 52–53
Testosterone, 50–51
Tetracycline, 82–83
Therapy. *See* Treatment
Thermography, 158–59
Thyroid malfunction and gout, 61–62
Time-release aspirin, 105
Tinnitus, 106
Toes affected in gout, 46, 48
Tolbutamide, Tolinase (tolazamide), interaction with sulfinpyrazone, 60
Tophi, 48–49, 51, 52–53, 55, 56–57
Toxicity of drugs. *See* specific medications
Tranquilizers, 95–96, 110–11, 143; interaction with alcohol and other drugs, 38, 59, 100
"Transference" folk theory, 11–12
Treatment: of dermatomyositis, 40–41, 113; of gout, 51–61, 107, 108; of osteoarthritis, 74–77, 104, 107, 110; of rheumatoid arthritis,

83–90, 92, 93, 108, 110; of scleroderma, 43; of spondylitis, 95–96, 107, 108, 110, 120, 122; of systemic lupus erythematosus, 33–38
Triamcinolone. *See* Corticosteroids
Tuberculosis, 3
Tylenol (acetaminophen), 59, 104

University of Manitoba, 152
University of Southern California, 65
University of Turin, 50
University of Wisconsin, 124
Uranium-ray hoax, 20
Urates, 47–48, 51, 52, 55, 56
Uric acid, 47–48, 55, 56–57, 61–62
Uricosurics, 56–60, 103
Urinalysis, 29, 88

Vaccinations, 92–93, 114
Valadol (acetaminophen), 59, 104
Valium (diazepam), 95–96, 110–11, 143
Vanquish, 104
Venereal infection, 3, 74
Vinegar as "remedy," 16
Viruses as possible causes of arthritic diseases, 29–30, 42, 82–83
Vision. *See* Eyes
Vitamins, 133–35; dangers of unneeded supplements, 60–61, 129, 134; as fad "remedies," 16, 135

Warfarin, interaction with gout medications, 60
Water retention, medications contraindicated in, 108
Weakness: in reaction to drugs, 58, 113; as symptom, 28, 39, 42, 80, 89
Weather, 84, 124–25
Weight: factor in gout, 52; factor in osteoarthritis, 64, 69, 76, 130; gain, in drug reaction, 108–9;

175